Natural
Medicine

NATURAL
MEDICINE

By

Robert Thomson

McGraw-Hill Book Company

New York · St. Louis · San Francisco · London · Mexico · Sydney · Toronto · Düsseldorf

2 3 4 5 6 7 8 9 0   FGRFGR   7 8 3 2 1 0 9

LIBRARY OF CONGRESS CATALOGING IN PUBLICATION DATA
Thomson, Robert, 1943–
   Natural medicine.
   Bibliography: p.
   Includes index.
   1. Naturopathy. I. Title.
RZ440.T47   615'.535   78-17598
ISBN 0-07-064513-2

Book design by Judith Michael

To my mother and the memory of my father

*Illness itself is one of those forms of experience
by which man arrives at the knowledge of God.
As He says, "Sicknesses themselves are My servants,
and are attached to My chosen."*

AL-GHAZZALI

Contents

Crisis • Adjustors • Ripening of Phlegm • Ripening Biliousness • Purgatives and Laxatives • Herbs to Provoke Emesis (Vomiting) • Diuretics • How to Apply Cupping

Notice

The information offered in this book is intended for practical application by physicians and members of other recognized healing professions. It may also have value to those engaged in research and education in the fields of natural medicine, herbology, and other related topics.

Persons who believe they are suffering from serious illness should consult a physician of their choice for diagnosis and treatment. In discussing the use of certain herbs and other procedures, we are not diagnosing or prescribing for any specific ailment, but only presenting the information for educational and scientific interest, without the author's or publisher's endorsement.

We cannot stress enough the necessity of using any information in this book only in cooperation with competent medical advice and guidance.

Foreword

No system of medicine has ever existed unchallenged. Rivalry among different schools of healing is an old tradition, as is medical heresy. Even when Hippocrates was teaching on the Greek island of Cos in the fifth century B.C., a rival school operated at Cnidus on the mainland.

The United States has been home to a number of unusual healing arts, some of which have grown quite strong. The first unorthodox system in America was Thomsonianism, the creation of Samuel Thomson, born in New Hampshire in 1769, and an ancestor of the author of this book. Samuel Thomson believed in healing by Nature, used herbs, followed a humoral system of medicine based on the teachings of Galen, and recommended steam baths to purify the body. Thomsonians were known as Steam Doctors or Steamers. One of their goals was "to make every man his own physician."

Mainstream American medicine has never been friendly to such challenges. Regular doctors persecuted the Thomsonians as they later persecuted, in turn, the homeopaths, osteopaths, and chiropractors. Yet other systems of medicine are more in evidence today than ever. Herbalists, acupuncturists, reflexologists, chiropractors, iridologists, and other "irregulars" abound and flourish.

Clearly, dissatisfaction with regular medicine is the major motivation behind increasing demands of patients for something different. The chief complaints against the orthodox system are that it is often harmful, often ineffective, and often too expensive. Modern hospital medicine is vulnerable on all three counts. It uses techniques and drugs that are productive of many adverse reactions, cost too much, and frequently do not cure.

It was Samuel Hahnemann, the founder of homeopathy in the late 1700s, who named regular medicine. He called it *allopathy,* from Greek roots meaning "other treatment," suggesting that it gave drugs on the basis of no particular logic, neither to counteract the symptoms of disease (antipathic medicine) nor to reproduce the symptoms of disease (homeopathic medicine) in order to mobilize the body's healing powers.

Allopathic practitioners did not like being labeled. After all, they thought they were the sum total of medicine and did not want to hear that theirs was merely one school of medicine. But the name stuck, and today, even though few homeopaths remain, regular doctors are still allopaths.

Sometime in the mid-1800s, when regular doctors and homeopaths were going at it tooth and nail, allopaths tried to redefine their new name in a more flattering way. They succeeded to some extent. If you will look up *allopathy* in a good dictionary, you will find two definitions. The first is Hahnemann's. The second gives a derivation from German roots meaning "all therapies" and identifies allopathy as a system of medicine embracing all methods of proven value in the treatment of disease.

That revisionist definition is a nice ideal. Why shouldn't practitioners use any methods that work, however peculiar they seem, if they do not harm? Unfortunately, modern allopathy does not begin to live up to that ideal. In my conventional medical education I heard absolutely nothing about acupuncture, manipulation, diet, fasting, herbal medicine, or any of many other methods I have since found to work and have a place in treatment.

In this book, Robert Thomson gives us a clear and practical presentation of a system of medicine that millions of people have used for many, many years. It is classical Persian medicine, based on the theories of Avicenna, which derive from those of Galen and the Greeks. Although this system—based on the body's four humours and an elaborate classification of foods, herbs, and diseases into categories of hot, cold, moist, and dry—reached its highest expression in Persia and Afghanistan, it is alive and well in many unlikely parts of the world. For example, Indians in remote areas of Mexico use a form of it, having learned it from their Spanish conquerors.

I must say here that I have very little experience with humoral medicine. I have never studied it carefully and do not use it in my own practice. Nor do I agree with all of its tenets. The idea that all disease originates with faulty digestion strikes me as dogmatic, for instance. And, although I am a great believer in the utility and safety of plant drugs as opposed to refined chemical drugs, I am unfamiliar with most of the herbal formulas given in the second part of this book.

Nevertheless, I am interested to know the details of a system of healing that has been a living tradition in so much of the world for so long, and I am impressed by Robert Thomson's own testimony of its effectiveness for him, his family, and friends.

For some years now I have paid attention to other systems of treatment. I have learned some interesting things. First, I have seen that no system has a monopoly on cures. Every school of healing cures some people some of the time. Even methods based on demonstrably wrong theories will cure some patients. Second, no system has a monopoly on failures. The most rational, scientific, "proven" form of treatment will not work at times. These observations suggest that whether a system of medicine works or not depends on factors other than its content. It appears to depend, especially, on a shared belief of patients and practitioners in the system and in each other.

In Afghanistan today, the natural medicine described here works for many people. It also exists in a cultural milieu that generates strong collective belief. Medicine in Afghanistan is much more allied with religion than medicine in America. The *hakims* or healers who practice it are often spiritually advanced individuals. The patients and practitioners who use this system follow styles of life and diet that may facilitate its effectiveness. Robert Thomson, who has lived among them, speaks their language, and admires their culture, believes in this kind of medicine and is able to make it work for him. Whether other Americans can make it work for them I do not know.

Allopathic medicine as it exists today has its place. It is good for treating major trauma and acute medical crises, especially of infectious diseases. The author of this book does not believe that allopathic treatment is worthless, nor does he negate the role of infectious agents in the development of certain illnesses. But in those areas where allopathy is weak—for instance, in the treatment of chronic disease, degenerative disease, allergies, and viral infections—natural medicine might be worth trying, particularly since it cannot do much harm on its own.

This book is important both as an academic treatise on Persian medicine in the twentieth century and as a practical manual of healing for those motivated to experiment with its principles. As an allopathic physician (in the best sense of the word) I am willing to be open-minded about any empirical system of treatment that works, as long as it is safe. In that spirit I recommend this book to all physicians and patients who wish to broaden their perspectives on medicine and health.

Andrew Weil, M.D.
Tucson, Arizona
Spring Equinox, 1978

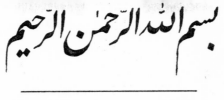

Introduction

The information shared with you in this book is my own humble effort to broaden the general knowledge of the public in the tradition of natural medicine. Some brief introductory remarks about how I came to write this book are necessary for you to understand my approach to the subject.

Five years ago, while pursuing a search for a usable, simple book on natural medicine, I read with great interest Alma Hutchens' *Indian Herbalogy of North America*. The book is based on impressively broad research and was the most useful treatise on herbs I had seen up to that time. I made an important discovery—one that led several years later to my writing this book. In her introduction, Hutchens mentions one Samuel Thomson (1769–1845), one of my distant ancestors, who himself was the first American of European descent truly to practice natural medicine in America, I learned. His system of healing is based upon the same principles of bodily balance that I had arrived at myself. I was lucky enough to obtain a copy of the original 1835 edition of his *Guide to Health.* This book, one of the most sensible ever written on herbology and natural medicine, contains many valuable and effective formulas. In addition to his own pioneering discoveries, Thomson made use of many American Indian remedies which he learned from the neighboring New England tribes. However, since Hutchens' book consisted mainly of generalized applications of herbs with few remedies for specific conditions, it did not entirely answer my purpose. Moreover, in the 150 years since Thomson wrote, there have been many advances in modern medicine that have shown aspects of his system to be inaccurate.

I knew from reading so many of the current texts that most of the information in them has been incorrectly adopted at random by today's faddists, with no regard for the time, manner, or place in which these remedies were originally given. I felt frustrated in my ten years' search of English-language books, because I could not find what I needed. Then, in 1975, I miraculously received a grant to study in the Near East for a year, and it was there that I made the discoveries which led directly to the writing of *Natural Medicine.*

In July 1975, my wife Ann and I departed for a year's residence in Kabul, Afghanistan—a city and country generally unknown in the West. In fact, I knew little about the country except for its long history of distinguished poets, philosophers, and musicians.

As our plane touched down at the small airport in the autumn dawn, we felt as though we were descending upon another age, something quite like descriptions in the Bible. The people, who turned out to be eminently hospitable, vigorous, and of good humor, were extraordinary and exotic in their baggy pants and turbans, and in those first few weeks we spent most of our time becoming adjusted to an entirely "other" way of life.

Part of the difference, we soon discovered, was in the food we were to eat. It was always delicious, healthy, and filling, but since no artificial fertilizers, herbicides, sprays, or additives of any kind are used there, we had to become acclimated to a different micro-life in the food we ate. The first signal was a rush of loose bowels for myself, and my wife seemed to be developing a serious cough with the early fall temperatures dipping to freezing in the six-thousand-foot altitude.

We both knew we would have to seek some kind of medical treatment, as I was without my own remedies due to the weight limitations on our flight over. We had to make a decision either to go to the United States Embassy's dispensary or to find a local healer (a course seriously criticized by our American friends). But by this time, having persistently studied Persian for several years, I was able to speak fluently with the local people, and I decided to ask an Afghan friend to recommend someone we could go to for treatment.

"There is a healer in Kabul," he told me, "who saved my life twice when I was a child. He's quite old now, but even so, he's considered the best doctor in the country."

My friend told me the healer's name was Hakim Sharif, which means "Exalted Healer," and gave us instructions how to get to his shop, which was located in the old bazaar. Inside the darkened shop, I first saw perhaps twenty men, women, and children lined up on both sides of a slightly raised divan upon which an elegant, aged man with a glowing white beard sat surrounded by several assistants. The walls of the wooden structure were lined floor-to-ceiling with bottles of many shapes and hues, and from the center of the room a wood stove cast a warmth over us all. There were also a dozen birds in cages— pigeons, rooks, thrushes, nightingales. I learned later that these feathered creatures had nothing to do with decor, but rather with the actual healing process.

We had been in the room only about a minute and were both transfixed with the scene, so much so that we didn't realize that everyone had stopped what they were doing to stare at these foreigners who must have accidentally stumbled into the Afghans' own medical clinic. I walked over to the healer and engaged in the customary extended greetings. He then told me to sit down at his feet, which I did. I was wondering how I could describe my symptoms of loose bowels without seeming rude or ridiculous in front of all those people.

To my surprise, Hakim Sharif asked me no questions at all about my ailment, but instead took my left hand and pressed the tips of his fingers to my pulse and felt the blood passing through the vessels for perhaps ten seconds. He then felt the tips of my fingers in the same manner. I concluded that he had made his general diagnosis and had found that my pulse was more or less normal. I again braced myself to answer the inevitable question about my ailment. But he asked nothing and instead reached to the shelf behind him for a small, round can and gave it to me. He told me to eat about a thumbnail portion dissolved in hot tea three times a day. Then he nodded and indicated that I was to go. Next it was my wife's turn. By now all of the people had gathered about us.

She sat down as I had done, and the healer once again asked

no questions but felt her pulse at the wrist and again on the tips of the fingers. The whole process took less than twenty seconds; this time, though, he called to one of his assistants to give her some pills, which was done, and the healer and everyone about us sat there waiting for us to leave. I asked how much the treatment cost, but he just shook his head slightly to indicate that I needn't pay. Knowing the small income of the people of this country, I began to insist until one of his assistants (who I later learned was his son) told me that if he had refused payment I would insult him by trying to press the matter.

On that first day of our visit we left, as I had no idea what else we could say to or ask of the man—and apparently nothing else was required for healing our illness. Both my wife and I, honestly, were leery of eating the substances he had given us until we found out what they were. So we returned to my friend who had directed us to the healer in the first place. He was glad we had gone, but a little surprised.

"What did he give you?" our friend asked. I showed him the small can and opened it, asking him what it was. "Oh, we all use this," he answered. "It's some kind of herbs ground up and mixed with ginger and honey." "Fine, but what's it for?" I asked. "When you have loose bowels," he said, "it balances your digestive system, which is what causes the problem with your bowels."

I said nothing further but immediately showed him the other medicine for my wife. He likewise knew this was a remedy for cough but did not know what specifically was in it—only that it worked.

My initial excitement at having made contact with a healer was increased over the following days, first of all because the remedies had worked: my stomach settled and my wife's cough disappeared. This seemed unusual in the extreme to me, not so much because we had been healed but because the *hakim* had made his diagnosis without either of us giving any clue at all to the nature of our illness. I was fascinated by a method of diagnosis that could so quickly and accurately pinpoint a specific ailment, almost without the patient knowing it.

Over the next twelve months I managed to become a friend and student of the Exalted Healer. For what he practiced was a rational system of natural medicine based on nearly 1400 years of tradition; this approach, if adopted in the West, would revolutionize the whole concept of medicine. I learned too that to become a healer in that tradition requires a long apprenticeship, usually thirty years, so the methods of treatment, diagnosis, and medical theory are hardly simple; they require decades of study. And the healer is not a fanatic, for there are several diseases he will not treat, such as tuberculosis, cancer, and certain types of internal disease too advanced for correction by herbs. In such cases, the patient is referred to a modern medical facility; this, however, is rarely needed, as the underlying principle of this system of medicine is one of prevention. The elements of diet, exercise, and prompt attention to any symptoms are behind the general good health of the population. One never sees obesity in that society, and cancer is practically unheard of.

The idea for *Natural Medicine* developed over the months as I went back several times each week to the Exalted Healer and watched him diagnose and prescribe natural botanicals for hundreds of different ailments. I began to cover other parts of the city and found the women who devote themselves to childbirth and the bonesetters, whose healing methods are said by the Westerners in residence in Kabul to be superior to the cast methods used in the West. I visited more than fifty shops that specialize in herbs from all parts of the globe. I spent an entire day with one herb seller who had more than 2500 different herbal remedies prepared and ready to dispense.

Still, though my collection of data was reaching large proportions, I lacked a unifying model upon which to write my book. Near the end of my stay, I finally found the key. Although Hakim Sharif had learned these methods from his own father, as he was teaching them to his son, he did say that there was a book called *Mizan-ul Tebb* ("The Basis of Medicine"). He thought it had been written several hundred years before; he wasn't sure. But he did say it was still in use today as the main reference work for practicing *hakims*.

Although the chances of finding this book seemed slim, I began a search for it. One afternoon, when I was making my usual rounds in the heart of the old city, I met yet another man who was selling herbs. I chatted with him for a while and finally asked if he knew where I could get a copy of the book. By happy chance, he had a copy, and after a great deal of haggling over the price he sold it to me. I immediately took it home and set about translating it, and as my work continued I enlisted the foremost botanical expert in Afghanistan to identify all of the herbs mentioned by the generic name. Surprisingly, nearly all of them are available in the United States.

There are millions of people today in America and other English-speaking countries who desire and are beginning to demand access to this traditional system of preventing illness and correcting bodily imbalance. Nearly all of the books written on this subject in the past decade are attempts to cash in on the nature fad, and many of the authors have no practical experience in the field they are writing about.

While compiling a subject listing recently for an encyclopedia of natural medicine, I was astounded to find the list topping the four-hundred mark. These were only the general categories, such as dietetics, hydrotherapy, naturopathy, Hoxsey Herbs, and so forth. If these were broken down into the various subcategories of individual diets and therapies, the list would run to over a thousand different natural modes. There is a present danger that natural medicine may fall victim to the same overcomplication that has plagued allopathic medicine, with many specialized vocabularies and disciplines. The time is ripe to take a look at natural medicine as a subject in itself, to look for the underlying principles and rules common to all the systems, so that in seeking any of these therapies, one can apply them against a *standard* of natural medicine.

I was struck by the fact that what I have been hearing about natural medicine in the United States is actually much more clearly and succinctly stated by these healers of old. They were perhaps less corrupt, and did not have to present theories in some strange linguistic judo to convince the reader it was something *new*. Most of today's health diets, or therapeutic diets, are simply variations of fasting. Some are mere gluttony. Would it not be better to return to the original concepts of fasting as evolved by people with more natural lifestyles? At least we should understand the basic principles of natural healing and admit that we did not invent them in the 1970s in the United States.

Thus, *Natural Medicine* is a compendium of knowledge gained from observation and study with the healers of the East, to which are added some contemporary practices in natural healing. It is my intention to provide a clear and simple condensation of the basic principles of natural medicine, along with some formulas utilizing harmless herbs to restore the human body to a balanced and harmonious condition. In so doing, I must admit at the outset a bias in favor of health in the sense that it is every person's normal and natural state, although we in this culture have come to accept a condition of our bodies which is far less than healthy, subnormal in nearly all respects. It is a cause of great anguish to witness the billions of dollars being spent on so-called remedies and cures, when in fact these are no more than efforts to blunt or remove the end symptoms of *causes*.

Natural Medicine comprises the essence of my own study over a period of nearly two decades and across four continents. In a sense it is also "Eastern," although that is perhaps an unfortunate word, for it is a system that has reached far into Western thought and behavior but was practically lost during the beginning of this century. The system I propose for men and women to follow is truly a *way of life*. In all of my observations, I have never found even one remedy that could be applied without the body itself being brought into play as the actual healing mechanism.

A growing number of allopathic physicians have grasped the need to apply more natural and complete means of treatment. Allopaths have generally had less faith in their own trade, and more faith in Nature, than is usually recognized—there are studies demonstrating that M.D.s and their families use less prescription drugs and have fewer operations than any demographically comparable group.

In addition, these allopathic physicians understand the need to apply more than chemical drugs and surgery in their treatments, and the ordinary people know they must accept individual responsibility for maintaining their bodies in health.

This requires, above all, persistent labor and attention to every act of each person's life. The fact is that natural medicine has survived for more than twenty-four centuries and is based on scientific principles that have been proved. Morever, this natural system is the basis of medical treatment for over half of the world's population *today*—in India, Pakistan, Afghanistan, Iran, Iraq, the Arabian Emirates, South America, much of Canada, and many such Western European countries as England, France, and Germany. Russia has a long and distinguished herbal history, as do Czechoslovakia, China, and other nations.

I have arranged the material into two divisions—the speculative and the practical. I begin with a brief history of natural medicine, which (although limited from a scholar's point of view) gives the general reader some idea of the origins and development of this tradition.

Next are given eleven principles of natural medicine, summarized from all the methods of healing I have studied. After this, a system of selecting and preparing foods according to their inherent qualities of heat and cold is explained.

In the second part, the Formulary, relying on my own education as a naturopath, naprapath, and herbalist as well as the information obtained in Afghanistan on traditional medicine, the causes, signs, and modes of treatment of various conditions of the body are given. In most cases, the following information is pointed out: (1) the general diagnosis of the character, causes, and signs of an imbalance; (2) any special diagnostic features; (3) general rules of treatment; and (4) the special methods of treatment by single and compound herbal remedies.

Every person who desires to learn this tradition of natural medicine will have to seek out knowledge in many places, for in the United States there is no place to attend for a formal curriculum of study.

However, as much as it is possible to learn some things from books, the lessons of natural medicine are, above all else, in Nature and must be learned directly from human experience, in the individual acts of daily life, whatever they happen to be.

A few brief words of thanks to people who helped me with

this work must be included. There are so many people I have learned from, often without their knowing; to them I owe greatest gratitude. Much of the material for this book was gathered while I was on a Fulbright research grant, which allowed me, for the first time in my life, an unrestricted and full period of time to devote myself totally to the study of spiritual and physical healing, without care or worry for my daily maintenance. Those who made this time productive by their help and encouragement included Larry Beck, Executive Director of the Afghan-American Educational Commission, and his staff, who often worked as though solely at my disposal. Professor Dannish Suljuki of the Faculty of Arts and Letters of Kabul University assisted me with the translations, which were true keys to understanding the basis of natural medicine; without his help this book surely would not have been written.

Dr. Louis Dupree and his wife Nancy both gave of their extensive knowledge of Afghanistan without promise of reward, and have my continuing gratitude. Dr. Richard Eaton of the University of Arizona first introduced me to the Persian language many years ago and spent many long (and I presume difficult) hours teaching me.

The people of Afghanistan lived up to their distinguished heritage of service to humanity. They are a rare people, who are loved by Nature. It is worth noting, I think, that our son was conceived one clear night near the birthplace of Maulana Jalaluddin Rumi, who gave to the world its greatest sequence of mystical poetry and whose name our son bears.

During several excursions into India, I was treated quite literally as a prince by the venerable Mirza W. D. Begg, who resides at the feet of the great saint Hazrat Khwaja Muinuddin Chishti and has devoted his entire life to the divine cause of love and peace. It was he alone who kept up my courage in the arduous study of the Science of Breath and other subjects essential to a mastery of the Natural Laws.

I must also acknowledge the assistance of many other persons who helped me with this book in their own way, among them Stephen Moore, M.D.; Robert J. Baumann, D.N.; Robert Martin, D.N.; Andrew Weil, M.D.; and Dr. Ludwig Adamec.

In Afghanistan, I offer my gratitude to the following persons and organizations: Pir Syed Daoud Iqbali, Shaikh Saleh Parvanta, Prof. Dr. Rahwan Farhadi, Nasratullah Laheeb, Hamayutallah Shahrani, Hassan Kamiab, Hon. Theodore Eliot, Ambassador to Afghanistan, and Dr. Jon Summers and his staff, Parvin, Younous, Zarghuna, Lahli, and Mohammad Jan.

A special grant was very deeply appreciated from The American Society of Kabul, which provided funds to complete vital translation work.

Martha Sowerwine and Harmony Noble extended themselves in the final editing and typing of the manuscript, and the fine anatomical illustrations were done by Cindy Lynn Cohen of the Department of Scientific Illustration at the University of Arizona.

I am especially appreciative of the help provided by my editor at McGraw-Hill, Fred Hills, who had the confidence to publish this book in the first place. Peggy Tsukahira, my manuscript editor, added many graceful improvements in the style and organization of the text to the benefit of the reader.

The Persian calligraphy that opens the Introduction is an invocation written in a stylized form, which is used by all *hakims* to commence any written work. It reads, *"Bismallah Ir-rahman, Ir-rahim,"* which means, "In the Name of Allah, Most Gracious, Most Merciful." It was drawn by Enayat Shahrani of Badakshan.

May God grant you Peace, Health, and Long Life.

Robert Thomson N.D., D.N.
(Hakim Moinuddin Chishti)

Tucson, Arizona
March 20, 1978

Part One

The Theory of Natural Medicine

Chapter 1

A Brief History of
Natural Medicine

The First Healers

Natural medicine has always been based upon a philosophy, and the first men in history to speculate systematically about the principle behind all things were the wise men of the East, who lived in the early part of the sixth century B.C. One of the most notable of these was Thales (c. 636–c. 546 B.C.), one of the Seven Sages of ancient Greece, who was born in Miletus and lived in the province of Ionia in western Greece.

Thales and his successors sought for the nature of man. In keeping with the prevailing religious and philosophical notions of their time they looked to the elements earth, water, air, and fire for an explanation and eventually developed a system based on the belief that all things were composed of a combination of these four elements and that individual characteristics of matter depend upon the proportion of each element.

A later thinker proposed that these elements joined together according to two principles that he called Love and Hate. Here, twenty-five hundred years ago, we have the origins of atomic theory and psychology in a nutshell. Alcmaeon of Croton, a young contemporary of Pythagoras, taught the necessity of physiological balance or harmony of the elements, which later led to Hippocrates' fundamental theory of the unity of the organism.

Hippocrates, often called the father of medicine, was born about 460 B.C. on the Aegean island of Cos to a long line of priest-physicians. Records indicate that he traveled widely over Greece, learning from others, and settled and was affiliated with the flourishing medical college at Cos. Hippocrates based his philosophy of health on the word *physis,* which meant simply "organism," or the organism in its unity. Unlike the earlier philosophers, whose intricate theories of existence had tended to separate man from his environment, sometimes even from his own soul, Hippocrates insisted that there was something greater than the organism—Life itself. He postulated that Life was comprised of a reciprocal relationship between organism and environment. In this constant interaction Hippocrates found the origin of disease. The organism grows at the expense of environment, taking from it what is necessary to sustain life and rejecting what is unnecessary. From Hippocrates' viewpoint, disease was the occurrence of severe difficulty in this digestion (*pepsis*) of the environment by the organism, or *dyspepsia.*

Hippocrates' popular reputation as the father of medicine is perhaps not entirely deserved, for, unlike several later physicians, he left no truly codified science; knowledge of him today rests chiefly on the code of medical ethics known as the Hippocratic Oath. The oath is recognized as having genuinely originated with Hippocrates, but the exact time and circumstances are not known. Here is the full oath:

THE HIPPOCRATIC OATH

I swear by Apollo the Healer and by Aesculapius, by Hygeia and Panacea, and by all gods and goddesses, making them my witnesses that I will fulfill according to my power and judgment this oath and this covenant. I will look on him who taught me this art as I do my own parents, and will share with him my livelihood. If he be in need, I will give him money. I will hold his offspring as my own brethren, and will teach them this art, if they wish to learn it, without fee or written bond. I will give them instruction by precept and by lecture and by every other mode to my sons, to the sons of him who taught me, and to those pupils who have taken the covenant and sworn the physicians' oath, and to none other besides. According to my power and judgment, I will prescribe regimen in order to benefit the sick, and do them no injury or wrong. I will neither give on demand any deadly drug, nor prompt any such course, nor, similarly, will I give a destructive pessary to woman. In holiness and righteousness I will pass my life and practice my art. Into whatever houses I enter, my entrance shall be for the benefit of the sick, and shall be void of all intentional injustice or wrongdoing, especially of carnal knowledge of woman or man, bond or free. And whatsoever, either in my practice or apart from it in daily life, I see or hear which should not be spoken of outside, thereon will I keep silence, judging such silence sacred. If then I fulfill this oath and do not violate it, may I enjoy my life and art and be held in honor among all men for ever; but if I transgress and prove false to my oath, then may the contrary befall me.

There is an additional line included in other versions that prohibits "cutting for stones," which means presumably to avoid surgery, leaving it to the realm of the "specialist."

There is no evidence that there was any compulsory enforcement of this oath; it existed rather as a code of the healing brotherhood, imposed upon students by the teacher. Its wisdom lies in its emphasis on the principle that the private life and ethics of a physician cannot be separated from his work with the sick. It also assumes a divine presence watching over the work of the physician, even though the invocation at the beginning of the oath reflects the influence of then-prevailing religious beliefs. Few, if any, physicians today claim allegiance to this oath.

As Ahmed Elkadi, M.D., commented in the September 1976 issue of the *Journal of the IMA*,[1] the contemporary secular codes of ethics, such as the pledges of the American College of Surgeons and the Geneva Declaration of Medical Ethics, compel the physician only to rely upon his own judgment by saying: "I pledge myself. . . ." In fact, the Hippocratic Oath was modified in Geneva in 1948, and, rather than eliminate the polytheistic gods of ancient Greece and replace them with the one-God concept of Christianity, they eliminated all reference to a supreme being of any kind.

The statement of avoiding carnal intent when entering the houses of the sick was also completely omitted in Geneva (although physicians are still sometimes criminally charged for ambiguous behavior during genital examinations). The Geneva Declaration also changed the direct forbiddance of inducing

[1] Islamic Medical Association, Pittsburgh.

abortion to "I will maintain with utmost respect the human life from the time of its conception."

Hippocrates had envisioned the ideal human organism as a whole being inhabited by a soul that was intimately tied to its environment, Nature. To this concept, the great physician Galen introduced the idea that humans could consciously influence the "use" of the environment for their sustenance.

Galen

Galen was born in 130 A.D., six hundred years after Hippocrates, at Pergamum, in northwest Asia Minor. This city in his day was culturally distinguished and had a renowned medical college, where Galen was introduced to medical subjects. He had been educated first in the sciences, philosophy, and logic at the insistence of his father, who decided when Galen was seventeen to add medicine to his curriculum. Then Galen spent nine years away from his birthplace, including a period of study at Alexandria, home of the most prominent medical college of the time.

Galen synthesized not only Hippocrates' work but all medical knowledge over the intervening six centuries. He felt that the force that pervades or inhabits the living organism was in fact a creative principle of being, which could use certain attractive, retentive, or expulsive faculties to promote development, growth, and nutrition. Also important among Galen's ideas were those of the modifying effects of food on the body, and that plants are affected by the soil they grow in and animals by their diet.

Next to *physis*, the most important factor in Galen's system is the *pneuma* or "vital air" through which the inherent powers of the *physis* become operative. The creative force itself is carried on the breath, originating in the action of the lungs; it is dispersed throughout the body according to natural principles and the needs of the body. He recognized that the *pneuma* traveled along specific paths to the heart and the brain and was conveyed all over the body by the network of nerves. Both

Galen and Hippocrates believed that there exist in the body various *humours,* which of necessity must be balanced equally in order for there to be a state of true health. Galen believed that all foods also contained their own characteristic humours, and thus an early dietetic system arose, similar in some respects to our concept of vitamins.[2]

Avicenna and the Canon of Medicine

After these underlying principles of natural medicine of Hippocrates and Galen there passed nearly nine hundred years without any significant development of medical theory. Modern medicine considers itself an outgrowth of the scientific rationale that developed especially forcefully in this century. Practically all of the nature-cure systems, on the other hand, as well as much of today's pharmacology is traceable to one man's influence. It is all the more surprising that this man is practically unknown in the West, as his medical theories and formulas are the basis of medical treatment for nearly half the world's population.

Abu Ali Al-Husayn ibn Sina, known in the West as Avicenna, was—in my view—the most illustrious physician in recorded history. He was born in 980 A.D. near Bokhara in present-day Afghanistan. Though that was the center of learning of the time, he had exhausted all teachers of the day by the time he reached his teens, and in fact explained logic to his master. He received no formal education in the sciences or medicine, but had physicians working under his direction at the age of fourteen.

He is perhaps less known for his medical genius than for his philosophy. His book *Kitab-ul-Ansaaf* (*The Book of Impartial Judgment*), in which, at the age of twenty-one, he answered 28,000 questions on theology and metaphysics, remains a significant and undisputed contribution to human thought.

Avicenna was extremely active in all realms of life, serving

---

[2] Arthur J. Brock, *Greek Medicine* (New York: AMS Press, 1972), pp. 9–39 *passim.*

several times as a court minister and on more than one occasion was caught up in intrigues that led him to flight or to prison. He wrote whenever he could—in prison, on horseback, or in the wee hours of the night after working all day. He wrote in verse to instruct his pupils, and produced important works on Sufi doctrines and behavior. He never had a library, and wrote primarily from memory. He is credited by scholars with an astounding outpouring of 276 works, touching on all aspects of human endeavor—medicine, natural history, physics, chemistry, astronomy, physics, mathematics, music, economics, and moral and religious questions. Among them is one of the greatest classics on medicine, the eighteen-volume *Qanun-i Tebb* (*Canon of Medicine*), which covers and orders all the medical knowledge of the world up to his time. The *Qanun* has maintained its authority through seven centuries of medical teaching and practice, and today remains the bible of medicine for practitioners in India (both Muslim and Hindu) and throughout the Near and Middle East. Large medical schools are devoted to teaching Avicenna's methods, and in India huge warehouse complexes are strategically located to supply the remedies from the *Qanun*.

Up to the end of the eighteenth century, the London Dispensary revealed considerable influence of the herbal remedies of Avicenna, and their use continued widespread into the nineteenth century. In fact, many of his remedies are still used in Western Europe and the United States, especially in rural areas that rely upon "home remedies." It remains for Western medical science to study this rich source of knowledge as one of the greatest systems of rational medicine ever devised.

Translations of Avicenna's *Qanun* remain incomplete and inadequate. A British doctor, Cameron Gruner, translated the first volume of the *Qanun* into English,[3] having been introduced to Avicenna's work by Hazrat Inayat Khan, a Sufi mystic from Hyderabad, India. The remaining seventeen volumes are available only in Persian and Arabic, with some translations into the Romance languages.

There is no question that considerable prejudice against all

[3] O. Cameron Gruner, M.D., *The Canon of Medicine of Avicenna* (New York: Augustus M. Kelley, 1970).

Muslim thought has existed in Europe and the United States up to the present time. However, the events of today's oil-crisis diplomacy are rapidly encouraging changes in attitude.

Natural Medicine is a first attempt to provide an introduction to the great medical thought and practice of Avicenna, taking these from the dusty backbins of scholars' shelves into the mainstream of popular use.

Recommended Readings

Browne, E. G. *Arabian Medicine.* Cambridge: Cambridge University Press, 1962.

Hall, Manley P. *Healing: The Divine Art.* Los Angeles: Philosophical Research Society, 1971.

Chapter 2

The Main Aspects of Healing

There is no lack of sound reasons for employing herbal medicines—or a natural system of living. The mission of this book is to revive these tenets of successful healthy human life. The road to health utilizing the great healing mechanism of nature—the human body—can be utilized by every person, although it may require a complete change of many established patterns of living.

What is Health?

We wish to approach health from an understanding of the nature of the human being as a whole, as opposed to the modern medical view of the body as a collection of separate parts, which can be assembled well or poorly according to heredity and environment. Natural medicine holds that *the body and soul form one complete whole.* This is similar to the holistic approach that has cropped up lately and underlies all natural systems of healing, but it is more: natural medicine assumes that all of the outward signs of hands and limbs, facial characteristics, hair color, eyes, skin, and all else are a reflection of a motive force *within*.

There is another aspect of the "whole" that causes us to view the internal organs and processes as interrelated; for example, the heart is not a single organ, but part of a "heart system" working within the body that affects points distant from the physiological heart. These *systems within* are called *humours*, and each must be in balance in terms of both temperature and moisture for there to be true health. The *hakims*, the physicians of the East, use a type of pulse diagnosis to determine how or where these internal systems have gone out of balance and from this choose a mode of treatment. The full concept of humours and internal systems will be presented in a later chapter, but the basis, the Code of Health of Nature, is based upon the twofold premise of *body and soul* and all the internal systems *as one whole*.

The great American physician Henry Lindlahr, one of the pioneers of natural medicine in the United States, stated in his *Philosophy of Natural Therapeutics*: "Health is normal and harmonious vibration of the elements and forces composing the human entity on the physical, mental and moral planes of being, in conformity with the constructive principle in Nature applied to individual life."[1]

The Eleven Principles of Natural Medicine

There are hundreds of books written by persons knowledgeable about healthy living. Every book on health or diet has its own maxims, some do's and dont's for proper living. There are, however, principles of natural medicine, which I have found repeated throughout the literature of natural medicine. These principles are essential, and without them health cannot be gained or maintained. Like all verities, they are simple to express, but difficult to apply and follow.

Principle 1: Enjoy Moderation in Work and Rest

So often there seem to be pressing reasons we cannot have the kind of job we want or cannot get "caught up on" our rest. But are any reasons valid when we know that prolonged abuse of the normal cycles of work and rest will lead to discomfort, pain, and disease?

[1] Henry Lindlahr, M.D., *Philosophy of Natural Therapeutics* (Chicago: Lindlahr Publishing Co., 1922), I, 23.

A young man came to fix an electric typewriter one day, and he had a rather pale complexion. I watched him work and got into a conversation with him. He had been raised on a farm in the Pacific Northwest and had been living in Tucson for about five years. He worked long days and had to wear a "buzzer box" around his waist to heed the beck and call of his employer. He confessed to me that he had been suffering from the most painful migraine headaches for nearly a year. He reported that he had gone to several doctors and had been prescribed Valium. Just the previous week, he had been to the hospital to have a full range of brain tests, but the doctors could find nothing wrong with him. I used a technique of ligamentous tissue massage on his neck, along with some techniques of balancing I had learned in the East, and within two minutes his headache had vanished. He was truly astonished, and kept bouncing his head and jiggling his neck to make sure the pain was really gone. This was merely a temporary relief, and he would have to make some major revisions of his dietary and work habits. He came to see me often over the next few weeks and was fully educated about the foods he was supposed to eat.

His headaches had left and did not return. I also advised him that the kind of work he was engaged in was not fit for most people, especially one who had the sensitive life of the open fields in his background. He took my advice, and after a serious talk with his family, decided to return to his family land in Oregon; the last I heard from him, he was a happy and balanced person. There are millions of people like this young man living lives that conflict with their own sense of self-worth, their own moral values, and keep such pressure upon them that they wonder what the purpose of life is after all. It takes great courage to uproot one's life, and there should be efforts made to do so in as smooth a manner as possible, with adequate planning. But, in terms of this first law, one must have a vocation that produces harmony of thought and action or one can expect to become ill in due time.

Another important point to remember is that for humans, the day is the time of work and night time is for rest and sleep. There are other millions of workers in factories and elsewhere who violate this most important law. While it may seem absurd to suggest so in the industrialized West, we should endeavor to go to bed shortly after nightfall and rise at dawn. This is Nature's law.

Principle 2: Moderation in Eating and Drinking

To those who have established a healthy life, to go about the streets and restaurants of any American city can only be a cause for pity. The basis of proper nutrition will be discussed fully in Chapters 3 and 4. Every method of natural healing involves greater or lesser degrees of fasting. Why? Because the body needs a complete or partial abstinence from food to bring it into balance from the effects of months or years of overindulgence. The comprehensive Tradition of Medicine of the Prophet Muhammad gives more emphasis to fasting and restricted diet than to any other factor. Moderation in drinking applies to the proper intake of any fluids. (By those seeking health, distilled spirits are shunned entirely.) For example, when milk or water is drunk with food, it dilutes the concentration of hydrochloric acid in the stomach, which can impair the full digestion of food. Partially digested food passes out of the stomach and places the burden of completing this process on other organs not designed for the primary digestive function.

Principle 3: Elimination or Evacuation of Superfluities

Charles Mayo once commented that in more than 10,000 operations on the abdomen, he never saw even *one* healthy colon. Another natural doctor in California reported that in twenty years of practice, he had seen only two x-rays of what could be considered "healthy" colons, the last one in 1953!

A young woman who came to me for health guidance had many complaints. "You have regular bowel movements, don't you?" I queried. "Oh yes," she answered. "Every other day, regular as clockwork," I noted. "Yes," she agreed. Then, I had to give her the news that a healthy body will produce a bowel movement on rising from sleep, after each meal, and before retiring. This is five movements per day! In her case, this meant that the toxic products of digestion and cellular metabolism were being kept in the body for forty-eight hours, when they should be expelled within six to eight hours. A considerable amount of reabsorption into the system occurs, so the body is required to be continually engaged in redoing the work it had already done.

The term *superfluities* does not mean only feces and urine; it also applies to mucus, sweat, and tears. These are all mechanisms for the body to eliminate matter unnecessary to sustain life and that, if allowed to accumulate, produce congestion of the eliminative system.

While I was studying natural medicine in Afghanistan, my teacher told me that the word *Afghan* also means a state, in a moment of purified emotions, when one is moved to tears. Persian poetry was born and raised in Afghanistan, and the people are very much moved by the exalted metaphors of their spiritual literature, so much so that it is not uncommon to see men and women sitting around after an evening of music and poetry weeping copious tears. This is a sign of health, to freely and spontaneously express all the human emotions, especially those of joy and compassion.

Principle 4: Dwelling in Regulated, Healthy Structures

Once I was traveling around Magdalena, Mexico, and rode in a truck out the back of town and came upon the people who work the rich fields there. I noticed that the people had erected small adobe houses in which little attention had been paid to niceties of style. Yet, alongside the dwellings, there were often expensive tractors and other farm machinery. These Mexican agriculturalists live *in and on the land* and consider a dwelling as simply sheltered quarters for sleeping and cooking.

There are no hard-and-fast rules for a building in terms of health, although from personal experience I have found those dwellings constructed of native earth to be most satisfactory in terms of maintaining a balanced temperature in many climates. There is a trend in the Southwest toward inexpensive modular homes, "mobile homes," that is very dangerous from a health as well as a safety standpoint. The concentration of negative metallic ionization around oneself drains off energy and affects the mind and body adversely by reversing polarity. If one must live in an apartment or house in a city, the minimum acceptable requirement is to have plenty of light, with a north exposure preferred. It is pathetic that we have shut ourselves off from Nature, and we have come to accept as a "natural" setting one in which a few houseplants are growing. Large numbers of the populace are fleeing to the Sun Belt of California, Arizona, and New Mexico for the clean air, sunshine, and humane life pace. In so doing they, of course, threaten the very things they seek by their numbers and initial insensitivity to the fragile balances that produce such excellent living conditions.

In short, it is best to spend as much time out of doors in Nature as possible and to utilize natural substances of earth and wood and cloth for sheltering the body.

Principle 5: Avoidance of Submission to Evil Things before They Become Uncontrollable, Stupendous, and Gruesome

One of the worst cases of abuse of this principle I have encountered was that of a woman in New York City. I was living in Kabul at the time a letter arrived from her, asking me for some kind of help—any help—for she sadly told me her entire life was "falling apart." I wrote her a letter of encouragement and promised to see her as soon as I returned. Upon arrival back in the States, I went directly to her home, which happened to be in Connecticut. In less than an hour, she told me a horror story of the gradual slipping away of all of her physical and emotional underpinnings. It had begun when she was first married nearly eight years before. Her menstrual periods began to cause her excruciating pain. She went to a doctor for treatment, and he told her it was her "nerves." She began drinking wine, often a half gallon during each night of her period. And another matter complicated her plight: she had little control over her bladder function, and she could not even go to the corner grocery store without having to stop and go into a restroom to relieve herself. The doctors prescribed various medications on which she relied to go to sleep, which lasted only a few hours regardless of what dosage of narcotics she took. In the past three years she had been to the top specialists in New York City, had twice had exploratory surgery, and had been told by the surgeon that she needed a hysterectomy to find relief. A definitive diagnosis of her problem was never made. Naturally, her marital life had degenerated; she was on the edge of insanity. Her arms and feet had lost all feeling. Yet her current doctor kept giving her prescriptions for Valium, Demerol, and so forth. Truthfully speaking, I thought she easily could be a suicide. She had no idea at all of why her problems had begun, whether they were physical or mental; and after going to so many physicians, she felt there was no hope. She was the epitome of one whose life had become "uncontrollable, stupendous, and gruesome."

This woman's complete recovery using the principles of natural medicine is practically a miracle. My response was to insist that she come with me to Arizona, which she did after several weeks of coaxing. We first of all put her on a strict regimen of proper nutrition, fresh vegetables, twice-daily laps in the pool, some light jogging, and—most important—a program of education about her own body. I enlisted the help of a natural doctor, who put her on an intense program of detoxification. After two days, the numbness in her arms and legs had disappeared; after three weeks, the periods that had maimed this woman's life had receded into a mild period of discomfort which was controlled by careful modified fasting for several days prior to menstruation.

Now, this woman was a very typical person, of average education, and one who had believed in doctors and that our national watchdog agencies would assure that the foods she was eating were safe and healthy. After her recovery to health, she no doubt knew more about healing than most physicians. Notice that I say *healing,* for health and its maintenance have nothing to do with diagnosis, but rather with a *way of life.* Not only had this woman been living a life at practical odds with health and sanity, but until she was provided some guidance, she had no idea whatsoever of how to get out of her predicament.

The real cause of her problems was that she submitted to many evil thoughts, especially those of self-doubt. She had also allowed her defenses against overuse of various dangerous drugs to slip until she was literally killing herself with medicines.

Medical doctors and skeptics may doubt this story, yet it is absolutely true. She is one of many who have straightened out their lives by returning to the natural laws of living.

Principle 6: Keep in Harmony All Psychological Ambitions and Resolutions

If one looks deeply enough into the subject, one can find that every disease originates in the mind. By this I mean that even though the immediate cause of disease may be improper diet over an extended time, one must accept responsibility for having consumed such foods. And the question then is *why* does a person eat things, or think thoughts, that are known to have a deleterious effect upon health? All religions, and especially the esoteric sides of religions, stress the overcoming of the ego, or appetitive soul. From this perspective, one must constantly be aware of the bad effects of wrong thinking, of stress, and of negative emotions. We know that worry, grief, and stress produce a toxin within the body. Those who follow the Christian Science teachings have obtained truly amazing results with the positive control of negative emotions. Dr. Edward Bach developed a healing system utilizing the essence of flowers to "cure" negative states of mind. His own reflections, *Heal Thyself*, are certainly worth careful application: "The abolition of disease will depend upon humanity realising the truth of the unalterable laws of our universe and adapting itself with humility and obedience to those laws." In other words, it is only through harmonizing the personality that healing of the body can occur.

The mind is essentially sustained by thoughts and imaginings. If one truly believes in the body and soul as one whole, it is obvious that the quality of this sustenance is of vital importance, and as much concern must be exercised over thoughts that are fed to oneself as over the food given to the body.

Principle 7: Acquisition of Silence Through Possession of Good Thoughts and Physical Exercise

It is a classic Eastern belief that silence is a characteristic of wisdom. And the wise men everywhere insist that real knowledge of God or Truth cannot be spoken of. Moreover, it is jarring to have someone around who always "shoots his mouth off." To see how difficult it is to keep silent, however, just arise one morning and consciously decide that you are going to be as sparing with words as you can. Usually, within a half hour, the decision is forgotten—until remembered in the midst of a babbling phone conversation or similar situation.

How many times have we said something that we wished we hadn't, and the desire not to have made a particular comment often disturbs one's mind for quite a time. It is easy to speak, but it is more difficult and requires will power to hold one's tongue. We can throw the breath out of balance by too much verbalizing.

The person who sits quietly throughout a long meeting and makes a comment at the end usually gets careful attention. It is a shock to hear words from one who is so silent; thus, the words are noted more carefully than if the person had been speaking through the entire meeting. People tend to ignore much of what is said by those who are usually labeled "blabbermouths," even though they may be well-motivated. It requires too much listening and thereby throws one of the senses of the listener—hearing—out of balance.

The suggestion of this principle is that the one who is able to measure his words does so through the means of cultivating cleanliness and good habits, and by regular exercise.

Clean habits means not only observing acute personal cleanliness but also keeping the mind focused on beneficial, harmonious thoughts. "A thought can sink a ship," it has been said. A jarring word or comment sets up a negative wave in the mind of the listener that can have repercussions down a long chain of additional encounters.

The reason physical exercise, vigorous exercise to the point of perspiration, is recommended to develop control over the mouth and thoughts is that such exertion forces the lungs to deep inhalation and expulsion in a balanced way. "He runs off at the mouth" is one of those observations that contains some truth, for, if the person truly understood this natural principle, he could "run off" the excessive words by actual exercise.

Control of the breath lies at the base of all systems of esoteric studies of spiritual advancement. "The first lesson is the breath, and the last lesson is the breath," say the Sufis, and it is only by consciously controlling the breath and its by-product, speech, that one can truly find contentment—the highest reward in life.

Principle 8: All Diseases Are Derived from One Chief Cause— Disorder of Rhythm

This principle has sometimes been given as the true essence of natural healing. Some call this the Unitary Theory of Disease. When I was writing this book, I sent a letter to a famous New York nutritionist, asking for his opinion on this theory. He wrote back that I needed a "high school course in biology," for, he informed me, everyone knows that diseases are caused by *germs*.

Yes, there are germs, bacteria, and viruses that bring about sickness, but not all people are susceptible to these pathogens. If they were, in any outbreak of epidemic disease, *everyone* who had contact with the disease would become ill—and everyone knows that some who are exposed do not fall ill. The reason for this is that those who are healthy are able to repel these disease-carrying organisms by means of their own bodily defense mechanisms.

In order to develop and maintain health, there must be rhythm. What does this mean? Our life is a constant process of activity, and we measure our amount of activity by means of the five senses—taste, touch, hearing, sight, and smell. The nature of activity is constantly to increase. This can be seen in the way a person begins walking with a normal pace, but as the destination comes closer, the pace of walking increases until the person may be literally running to get somewhere.

The same is true with sight. The eyes look at dozens of things each day with a purpose in mind. But the eyes also view hundreds, or thousands, of sights without meaning to do so. This not only involves much waste of energy, but leads to disharmony of the sense of sight. The reason may be a headache, which is a signal to the mind to quit looking at things, to rest. While there are many other causes of headache, no doubt this overstimulation of the sight faculty leads to many cases of headache. The cure, obviously, is to rest the eyes.

Normal activity stimulates and builds up the body, but in our culture, there is far too much emphasis placed upon activity and little or no thought given to relaxation and rest. The mystics spend much more time in repose than in activity, for they know that harmony comes only from the power of the mind to control activity.

There are many means for controlling the physical senses, and a person's age, sex, general physical health, and other factors will determine which is best. But a person who tries to develop health without bringing the sense under control will have no success.

Principle 9: A Perfect State of Health Arises from a Proper Balance of the Temperatures of the Four Elements: Earth and Water (fluids and solids) and Fire and Air (activators)

It must be remembered that heat is life, and cold, death. A good illustration of this point is that molecular activity speeds up when heated and slows when cooled. Samuel Thomson based his entire healing system upon this idea. The construction and organization of the human frame, in both men and women, is essentially the same, being formed of the four elements: earth and water constitute the solids of the body, which are made active by fire and air. Heat in a particular manner gives life and motion to those elements; and when this heat is extinguished from whatever cause by the other elements, death ensues. Thus a perfect state of health arises from a due balance of the temperature of the four elements. When this balance of temperature is by any means impaired, the body is more or less disordered. In the chapter on disease, it will be fully explained how the body uses an exceptional and intense heat—a welling up of the essential life force—to repel disease.

Principle 10: Food Is Transformed into the Life Force of Heat by Digestion; Disease Follows when Food Is Not Digested Properly

Food taken into the stomach, in being digested, nourishes the system and produces the heat on which life depends. However, constantly eating too great a quantity of food (or food altered by chemicals and unsuitable for nourishment) causes the stomach to become foul, so that the food is not properly digested. An overload of food causes the digestive powers to be thrown off, not only in the stomach but all along the digestive system. This in turn allows the force of cold to take the upper hand, so to speak. Fever is no more than an artificial heat produced by the body in an attempt to restore this balance.

Principle 11: Fasting Is the Best Medicine

The Prophet Muhammad ordered fasting for thirty days each year for his followers. The Lord Jesus likewise commanded his people to fast to recover health. The purpose of this divine wisdom is to allow the organs and processes of the body a chance to rest and recover from the overload of much food or improper digestion. All forms of natural healing utilize some form of total or modified fast. This final principle is perhaps the most common of all methods for recovering or maintaining health, and so will be discussed at length in Chapter 5.

According to the true principles of natural medicine, as practiced for 2500 years, the balance of the elements or humours of the body lies at the base of maintaining health. With the foregoing eleven principles as a basis for natural health, let us look at them more closely and learn the specific methods of putting them into practice as a way of life.

Recommended Readings

Bach, Edward. *Heal Thyself.* London: C. W. Daniel, 1974.

Boyd, Doug. *Rolling Thunder.* New York: Dell, 1974.

Khan, Hazrat Inayat. *The Sufi Message of Hazrat Inayat Khan,* Vol. IV. London: Barrie & Jenkins, 1972.

Szekely, Edmond Bordeaux. *The Essene Science of Life.* San Diego: Academy Books, 1975.

Thomson, Samuel. *Guide to Health; or Botanic Family Physician.* Boston: J. Q. Adams, 1835.

Chapter 3

On the Origin of Illness

Food

"It should be known that the origin of all illnesses is in food." This is the claim of the latest natural medicine practitioners, and has been the cause of much debate and of vehement denials by large segments of the commercial food industry. The source of this quotation is a text on the philosophy of history, written by the Arabic philosopher Ibn Khaldun in 1377—six hundred years ago. This points up part of the problem with the present-day food faddists, who are rushing out so much "new" information that it cannot be comprehended or ordered by the average person. We need to understand, in a simple way, just what the body goes through in maintaining itself.

The Stomach Is the Home of Disease

"The stomach is the home of disease. Dieting is the main medicine. The origin of every disease is indigestion." These statements are from the Comprehensive Tradition on Islamic Medicine of the Prophet Muhammad, written more than fourteen hundred years ago.

"The stomach is the home of disease" means that this is where disease is born, is nurtured and thrives. "Dieting is the main medicine": dieting means going without food; thus hunger (or fasting) is the greatest medicine, the origin of all medicines.

"The origin of every disease is indigestion" can be understood in that indigestion is the addition of new food to food already in the stomach before it has been digested.

The Process of Digestion

Humans preserve their life through nourishment, which they obtain through eating. The digestive and nutritive powers are applied unconsciously until the food becomes blood, and then the growing power takes over and turns it into flesh and bones. Digestion means that the nourishment is changed inside the body by natural heat (boiled, or "cooked") until it actually becomes a part of the body.

The food that enters the mouth and is chewed by the jaws undergoes the influence of the heat of the mouth (from the body temperature) and the action of enzymes that cause chemical reactions, which again cause heat.

The food is then swallowed directly into the stomach, and the heat of the stomach (hydrochloric acid) boils it further, until it is a semi-fluid mass called chyme—that is, the essence of the boiled food. The stomach sends this essence on to the liver, and that part of the food that has become solid sediment is ejected in the bowels, through the urethra and rectum. Once these sediments are rejected, the chyme is more refined, and the heat of the liver then boils the chyme further, until it becomes fresh blood. On this blood there swims a foam which results from the boiling, called yellow bile. Parts of this, as the process continues, become hard and dry and are called black bile. The natural heat of the liver is not quite sufficient to boil the coarser parts left, which are called phlegm. The liver then sends all of these parts into the veins and arteries, where the natural heat again begins to boil them, continuing the process of digestion. The pure blood generates a hot and humid vapor (called in natural medicine the blood humour) that sustains the animal spirit in humans. The growing power acts upon the blood at this stage, and it becomes flesh. The thicker parts of it become bones. The parts the body does not need or cannot use (the by-products or waste) are eliminated as the various kinds of excesses—such as sweat, mucus, saliva, and tears.

While the foregoing is not a full and scientific explanation of all that transpires in digestion, it is what does happen, stated in terms that can be comprehended by anyone.[1]

The Signs of Illness

The first sign of most illnesses is fever. Fevers occur when the body's natural heat is not able to complete the process of boiling in each of those stages. The nourishment is thus not fully assimilated. Usually, the reason for this is either that there is a great amount of food in the stomach and it becomes too much for the natural heat (or, the body is not producing enough hydrochloric acid) or that more food is put into the stomach before the process of boiling the first food has been completed. In this second case, one of two things happens: either the body ignores the first food—in a half-boiled state— or it splits its heat and half-digests both of the foods. In either case, the heat is insufficient to complete the process at this stage.

The stomach sends the food in this state to the liver, which likewise is not strong enough to assimilate it fully. Often the liver *already* contains unassimilated food which has been sent to it. The liver sends all of it to the veins in an unpurified state.

When the body has received what it needs to sustain itself, it eliminates the unassimilated excess, along with the natural excess, such as sweat, tears, mucus, and so forth—if it can. But often the body cannot expel all of the unassimilated superfluities arising from overeating or wrong foods, containing chemicals which the body is not designed to digest. This unassimilated excess remains in the veins, the liver, and the stomach and increases with time. Any composite humid substance that is not boiled and assimilated undergoes putrefaction. Such putrefaction may occur in any limb, organ, or other site in the body. Then a disease will develop in that place, or the body will be affected in principal limbs or organs, because that organ is ill

[1]Ibn Khaldun, *The Muqaddimah*, trans. by Franz Rosenthal, ed. and abridged by N. J. Dawood. (Princeton, N.J.: Princeton University Press, Bollingen Series, 1967), pp. 386ff.

and produces an illness of its own powers. This covers all illnesses; their origin as a rule is in the food. Consequently, the unassimilated nourishment becomes putrid. Anything in a process of putrefaction generates heat, and this heat is what, in the human body, is called fever.

We can understand quite simply how this process operates in the case of the "common cold." The origin of the cold is in digestion, or lack of it, and when there develop superfluous matters in the body, a disturbance is caused in the particular organs. The body attempts to deal with the faulty digested matter, and even sends other organs to pitch in to help. But the body cannot keep this up, especially if no measures are taken to relieve the body of accumulated matter. The process slows down due to the excess matter, and remains in the stage of phlegm. This adds further congestion, until such a point is reached that there develops the heat of a fever, which accelerates the digestion of the food by cooking it with this intense heat. Once it is sufficiently "cooked," the body can excrete it, and does so copiously in the form of excretions from the nose, mouth, and eyes. The reason that the body so often contracts colds in the wintertime is that there is further lowering of the innate heat of the body from lowered outside temperatures, by a lowering of the internal temperature by breathing in cold air and similar effects of cold climate.

This points up the folly of attempting to "control" or stop a cold, for by doing so one only assures that the congestion and accumulated superfluous matters will be driven further into the body and eventually seriously undermine the functioning of major organs. The correct treatment is to assist this entirely beneficial process of Nature, to assist the development of inner heat and the elimination of excess phlegm.

Fevers are the main sign of illness. Some fevers can be cured by not giving a sick person any food for a certain period of time. The body knows this instinctively; the desire for food is automatically interrupted during the first signs of illness. But we often think that food is necessary during a fever, and try to feed a sick person. This is working against the body's innate knowledge of how to heal itself! Once the fever has ended, the proper nourishment must be taken until the person is completely cured. In a state of health, it is obvious that proper nourishment is the best and only "preventive" medicine there is.

Our own little son, when he was a year old, developed teething pain. His body decided that he shouldn't eat, and he refused all food. But we worried about his getting enough food, so we kept him on a liquid diet of raw cow's milk. After three days of this, we were jolted with alarm to hear him screaming in his bed. We rushed in to find that he had vomited his "nourishment," and that the milk had become puttylike chunks. I felt his head: he had a fever. He kept this fever for the next two days, and refused all food, but did drink water— Nature's greatest tonic and cleanser of the kidneys. What had happened, from the natural medicine point of view, is that drinking so much milk had caused an overabundance of phlegm in his body; his digestion then said "Stop! No more!" and his internal mechanism developed a fever, to boil the phlegm and expel it. If we watch the health processes of small children and infants, we can often learn how Nature works in ideal ways.

Disease and Environment

The incidence of illness is most frequent among people who inhabit settled areas, in cities, because they live a life of luxury and excess, or, in some cases, due to the press and ills of humanity, they are cast into a life of poverty and want and lack adequate nourishment. Also, they are exposed much more frequently to germs.

They exercise little or no caution in the foods they eat, and they prepare their food, when they cook it, with a mixture of too many things, such as spices, herbs, and fruits, both fresh and dried. I saw one cookbook, published in New York, that had a recipe for a dish which contained more than twenty-five kinds of vegetables, fruits, and meats. This kind of nourishment does not often agree with the body and its parts.

Moreover, the air in cities is putrid and corrupt, due to the mixture of various industrial wastes in it. Pure air gives energy to the spirit and strengthens the force of heat upon digestion. Corrupt air corrupts digestion.

People should dwell in rural areas, get their foods in natural form from the earth, and not use any artificial means to grow them. They should restrict their diet to foods that are in season in their particular locale. They should eat on a schedule and keep their routine according to natural cycles. The air should be free from impurities. Their food should be taken plain. Exercise—by working in fields, riding horses, going hunting—is necessary. In this way of life, digestion is very good, and as a result, the need for medicine is little. One's temper is healthier. Perhaps this is one reason that physicians are practically never to be found practicing among rural peoples. If they could find livelihood, they would be there.

The Doctrine of the Four Elements

All systems of natural medicine speak of the four elements we gave in Principle 9. Two of these are light (Fire and Air), and two are heavy (Earth and Water). In terms of qualities, the light elements are weak, positive, active, Heaven, and male (because it is conferring or inceptive). The heavy elements are strong, negative, passive, Earth, and female. We do not mean, let us quickly note, that men are "weak" and women "strong," but rather that the ionic charge for the light elements is positive, and for the heavy elements the charge is negative.

In fact, symbols of the religions of the world are composed of this archetype: in the cross of Christianity, there is the negative pole lying horizontally, representing Earth, or the Mother, which is *made positive* by addition of the vertical bar of male or activator. All humans are borne by the female, but she could not produce without the complementary force.

Earth

Earth is an element usually situated at the center of our existence. In its nature it is at rest, and all other elements gravitate toward it, however far away they may be, because of its inherent weight. It is cold and dry in nature, and it appears so to sight and touch, so long as it obeys its own nature and is not changed by any other agency. It is by means of the earth element that the parts of our body are fixed and held in place; thus the outward form of the body is due to this earth element.

Water

Water is a simple substance whose position in nature is exterior to the sphere of the Earth, and interior to that of Air. This position is due to its density relative to Earth and Air. It is cold and moist in nature. The purpose of Water in the scheme of Creation is that it is easily dispersed, and thus assumes any shape without permanency. In the construction of "things" it allows the possibility of their being shaped and molded and spread out. Shapes can readily be made from it, and just as easily dispersed. The dry elements, on the other hand, can be made into forms only with difficulty, and also dispersed with difficulty. When dryness and moisture alternate, the former is overruled by the latter. Moisture protects dryness from crumbling (as moist earth, or mud) and, likewise, dryness prevents moisture from dispersing. Thus they are interacting and interdependent.

Water is absolutely essential to life. The *Quran* says specifically: "The parable of the life of this world is like *water* which We send down from the cloud so the herbiage of the earth become luxuriant *on account of it* [18.45]."

Air

Air is an element whose position in Nature is above Water and beneath that of Fire due to its relative lightness. In Nature it is hot and moist, and its purpose in Nature is to make things finer, lighter, and more delicate and thus more able to ascend into higher spheres. It is also the agent by which breath moves in and out of the body and causes or makes possible the involuntary movements of the body.

Fire

Fire is also a simple substance, situated higher than the other three elements; it reaches to the Heavens. It is hot and dry in Nature, and its role in Creation is to rarefy, refine, and intermingle all things. It has the power to penetrate and can ride through the element of Air. It has the capacity of overcoming the coldness of the two cold, heavy elements, Earth and Water, and so creates and maintains harmony among the elements.

According to the systems of the ancient physicians, each element has a corresponding humour in the body: the black bile humour relates to Earth, the phlegm humour to Water, the blood humour to Air, and the yellow bile to Fire. The chart on page 40 portrays further attributes of the elements as they correspond to aspects of human physiology.

All natural qualities arise from the various combinations of the four elements according to the laws of action, and with the dominance of one or more of them, we can expect corresponding strength of the bodily systems. Not only the physical systems of the body, such as liver function, breathing, and so forth, but also emotional makeup, character, and even talents for crafts and music, literature, or politics are all colored by the dominant element. Thus the study of a person's features, gestures, voice, posture, hands, and other characteristics acquires an added meaning and informs us about the relative strength or weakness of the various systems of the body.

According to natural law, the elements are always in constant flux within the human being. The changes are the important thing. We tend to notice the outward form and to ignore the process of change that is always taking place. The *hakims* teach that "things" in themselves exist only as a function of God's constantly acting creative power. If He suspended that power, all would instantly cease to be.

As Cameron Gruner pointed out, the metaphor of a dance is most appropriate. There is the total event, or act: the dance. In reality, it is *composed* of an infinite succession of "points," which we can easily see by means of photographs. It is only the life force dancing through the human body that makes this a

Element	Tendency	Bodily system	Excretion	Sense	Bodily function	Mentality	Mental state
Earth	Spreading	Skeleton	Feces	Touch	Form	Torpid	Obstinacy Fearfulness
Water	Drooping downward	Muscles	Urine	Taste	Nutrition	Phlegmatic	Submission Affection
Air	To and fro	Circulation Skin	Saliva	Hearing	Respiration	Cheerful	Humor
Fire	Rising	Liver	Sweat Tears	Smell	Digestion Voluntary movements	Emotional	Weeping or Anger

(Adapted from Gruner, *The Canon of Medicine of Avicenna*)

human "life"; without it, all that is left is the lifeless images upon paper.

The growth of seeds displays this same phenomenon. The Sun, by means of its power of heat, penetrates the Earth and by means of a succession of shocks or signals to the seed, informs the seed's germinal center to commence a series of acts of its own. The Earth and Water elements in the seed are acted upon by the Air and Fire elements in a way that produces starch; further interplay of these two forces causes a further change into glucose, and thus a shoot springs up, and rootlets begin to penetrate the earth, searching for Earth and Water while the leaves rise upward, seeking Air and Fire.

This explanation describes the action of the imponderable elements, whereas the physiologist works out these changes in terms of the material chemical elements. The former views the matter with "faith," and the latter with faith in the material only. While the Doctrine of the Elements has been scorned by modern science, it nonetheless remains the world view of billions of souls upon earth and, often, even extended education in the structure of Western academics does not displace this conception.

The Doctrine of Temperament

The continuous process of this transforming of potentialities into actualities is what we call *temperament*. It results from the interaction of the four contrary qualities residing within the elements, heat, cold, moisture, and dryness.

The four qualities combine in pairs in four ways: hot and dry, hot and wet, cold and dry, and cold and wet. Widely divergent things, such as seasons, life stages, secretions of various bodily organs—as well as food—are classified according to these qualities.

In most of the world where this system is in use, one finds much more application of simple hot and cold qualities than of the compound qualities. The male is considered hot and the female cold. Because of this assignment, a woman who gives

	Hot and wet	Hot and dry	Cold and dry	Cold and wet
Season	Spring	Summer	Autumn	Winter
Age	Childhood	Youth	Maturity	Old Age
Region	East	South	West	North
Element	Air (steam)	Fire	Earth (dust)	Water
Humour	Blood	Yellow Bile	Black Bile	Phlegm
Temperament	Sanguine	Choleric	Melancholic	Phlegmatic

birth to a son is considered to have hot milk; if a daughter is born, the mother's milk is cold.

Individuals with light complexions are thought generally to be cold in nature, and those with darker skins are hot. Color differentiation also forms the basis for most plant classification: plants that produce white flowers are usually cold, while those with colored blooms are hot.

There are several ways in which temperament can become dominated by one factor or another. Whenever the four elements are not in a state of equilibrium, there is a state called *intemperament*. The kinds of intemperaments are:

Hot intemperament: temperament hotter than it should be, but not moister or dryer.

Cold intemperament: colder than it should be, but not moister or drier.

Dry intemperament: drier than it should be, but not hotter or colder.

Moist intemperament: moister than it should be, but not hotter or colder.

These four conditions are *simple* intemperaments, and last momentarily before leading to a *compound* intemperament. For example, when the body becomes too hot, the body also becomes drier than it should be, because heat dispels moisture.

The relative degrees of inherent temperament are given below:

In degree of heat:

1. Breath   (Hottest)
2. Blood
3. Liver

4. Flesh
5. Muscles
6. Spleen
7. Kidneys
8. Walls of arteries
9. Walls of veins
10. Skin of palms and soles   (Least hot)

In degree of coldness:

1. Phlegm humour   (Coldest)
2. The hairs
3. Bones
4. Cartilage
5. Ligaments
6. Tendons
7. Membranes
8. Nerves
9. Spinal cord
10. Brain
11. Fat
12. Oil of the body
13. The skin   (Least cold)

In degree of moisture:

1. Phlegm humour   (Moistest)
2. Blood
3. Oil
4. Fat
5. Brain
6. Spinal cord
7. Breasts and testicles
8. Lungs
9. Liver
10. Spleen
11. Kidneys
12. Muscles
13. Skin   (Least moist)

In degree of dryness:

1. Hair   (Driest)
2. Bone
3. Cartilage

4. Ligaments
5. Tendon
6. Serous membranes
7. Arteries
8. Veins
9. Motor nerves
10. Heart
11. Sensory nerves
12. Skin   (Least dry)

The innate heat of the body begins to dissipate after middle age, because the air surrounding all the body dries up the moisture. The innate heat itself assists in this drying process, as do all actions of the body involving effort. Thus the innate moisture of the body must eventually come to an end. When it does, the faculties are completely unable to function, and death occurs. The duration and continuance of life depends on this inherent moisture, which is affected most negatively by ill-digestion of food or harmful excesses.

The normal temperament of youth is hot, and in the last stages of life it is cold. That moisture is predominant in youth is due to the growing process and evidenced by the softness of bones. Old people are not only colder in temperament but also drier, as shown by the brittleness of their bones.

The reason that females live longer than males is that they are inherently moister than men. They are also colder, which is why they are smaller, as their inherent heat is not sufficient to produce tall growth.

In natural medicine, the interplay of these temperaments and intemperaments is carried on or manifested in what are called humours, which can be described as bodily fluids (although not all bodily fluids are humours; for example, urine is a fluid but not a humour). To understand the application of herbal preparations to the inharmonious conditions of the body, it is first necessary to understand the nature of food and the body in terms of these humours—for, in applying herbs, one is simply introducing various amounts of concentrations of these temperaments and humours.

Recommended Readings

Bailey, Alice. *Esoteric Healing.* New York: Lucis Publishing Company, 1967.

Gibbings, Cecil. *Divine Healing.* The Hague: East-West Publications, 1976.

Khan, Hazrat Inayat. *Healing.* Tucson: Ikhwan Press, 1975.

Leslie, Charles. *Asian Medical Systems.* Berkeley: University of California Press, 1976.

The Medical Group, Theosophical Research Center, London. *The Mystery of Healing.* Wheaton, Ill.: The Theosophical Publishing House, 1968.

Wendel, Paul. *Standardized Naturopathy.* Brooklyn, N.Y.: Paul Wendel, 1951.

Chapter 4

Temperature-Balanced Food: The Humoral Diet

Hot and Cold

Today, the treatment of disease by means of food is coming to the fore. This is usually done by noting the food value of substances eaten—such as the amounts of various fats, protein, carbohydrates, vitamins, trace minerals, and so forth they contain, and adjusting the diet according to what is deemed best for the specific disorder. The method of natural medicine is to determine the physiological and psychological incompatibilities of each component of the person's diet and to select various articles of food according to their inherent nature, so they will be in harmony with the person consuming them.

The healers of Afghanistan considered many factors of a person's environment before suggesting a diet. For example, they might note the local barometer, thermometer, humidity, hours of sunshine, wind direction and velocity, the character of the immediately preceding season, clues offered by migration of insects, rodents, and birds, presence of certain kinds of parasites, and many other factors.

The quality of food determines quality of chyme produced, which determines the quality and amount of the four humours. This in turn determines the quality and quantity of the waste products or superfluities, and these excesses affect the free flow of life juices through the body. Thus, a diet can be based upon a harmonizing of the four humours in the body, by selecting foods whose innate character is hot or cold, according to the temperament of the individual. (The closest similar mode used today would be classification according to acid and alkaline).

The facing table gives the values for many common foods.

46

	Hot	Cold
Meat and fish	mutton fish chicken eggs liver (all kinds)	beef goat (female)
Dairy products	clarified butter cream cheese sheep's milk cream (even cows' milk)	cow's milk buttermilk yogurt dried cow cheese butter cheese (except cream cheese) refined butter
Vegetables	onions leeks eggplant chickpeas red pepper green pepper carrot seed squash	potato tomato cucumber lettuce carrots all pickled vegetables legumes: beans, peas, lentils turnips
Fruits	mulberries red raisins green raisins olives ripe grapes pomegranates all dried fruits pumpkin	watermelon lemons oranges unripe grapes
Nuts	almonds pistachios pits of fruits (e.g., apricot kernels) walnuts pine nuts	
Other foods	thin-grain rice white sugar brown sugar	thick-grain rice rock candy
Beverages	black tea	green tea
Herbs	saffron cardamom rue mint anise	dill henna
Other	all modern medicine sweet things	bitter things sour things

Since, according to humoral theory, particular diseases are the result of excess of heat or cold in the body, it is easy to see why efforts should be made to balance the diet according to the values of each food, especially in relation to age, environment, physical factors, and so forth. For example, children (who are very hot) often get sore throats or coughs in summer (hot season) from eating greasy foods (hot). Thus it is simple to see that to avoid sore throats and symptoms of a "summer cold," one should keep children from eating greasy foods. A winter cold is likely to be caused by cold weather, therefore sour things such as pickles (cold) should be avoided.

In general, when people are ill, the hotter (richer) foods should be eliminated in favor of more easily digested foods.

The Ideal Diet

Many people desire a "once-and-for-all" diet, a strict list of each food to be eaten at precise times to assure good health. But our bodies are constantly changing, by time of day, by age, by season, by varying stages of health, by mental moods, physical exertions, and other factors; thus there is no one diet that can be said to be appropriate to all people at all times. Nevertheless, we can identify certain principles of eating which give a stability to our human organism and provide the most reasonable expectation of maintaining health over a period of time. Among the Muslims, the single most significant factor of dietary regimen is the inclusion of total fasting for one continuous month each year. This period of fasting, called Ramadhan, is part of religious law, and no one intentionally ignores it. In America, some have relegated the fasting to the province of the kook, and only those who are truly fanatic would imagine abstaining from all foods. Yet this is exactly what our bodies need to recover from the abuse which has been overworking the normal functions. I know a man in San Francisco who enjoys excellent health, who regularly fasts one day each week, a program recommended by many fine natural nutritionists. Fasting will be discussed in detail in the next chapter. For now,

I wish to present some general regulations in regards to food and drink.

Mealtimes   Ordinarily, there should be three mealtimes each day. Breakfast means literally "breaking of the fast" of the prolonged period the body has gone without food during the night—a natural fast, if you will. This should be a substantial meal of some kind of whole-grain bread, fruits, eggs or cheese, and tea. The time for breakfast is just after rising from sleep, after bathing and any prayer or meditation. Dinner is taken just after the sun passes its zenith in the sky, and its composition will largely depend on the kind of work one does, season, and so forth. The main meal is supper, taken just after sunset; this meal should include meat or vegetable protein, wheat or other whole grains, carbohydrates, fats, and salts.

Eat food in season   When eating in Afghanistan, we had all manner of fruits and vegetables, but not all year long. We arrived in the fall, and so we had the full array of vegetables, which were very large and of full flavor and texture without being pithy. The melons were just on the market after the heat of late summer. But after about a month of this wealth, our cook simply wasn't serving so many different varieties of vegetables; he informed us that their season had ended. There were other treats even in winter, such as the sudden appearance of blood oranges, along with very rich and sweet pomegranates. Of course, we were less active in winter, and stayed indoors more, and so our diet was rightly being changed by nature to be in line with the normal seasonal changes forced upon our habits. Since Afghanistan was a so-called backward country, with undeveloped transportation systems and no industry for preserving foods, we *had* to eat only what was in season. It took a little adjusting to, but back in the United States and living in the Southwest, we found that our diet was more beneficial when we followed the growing seasons for our locale and resisted the temptation of buying processed and preserved foods trucked in to the supermarkets from as far away as Florida.

Do not eat unless hungry A person should not eat unless there is a true and ready appetite. When the appetite comes, the meal should be consumed soon, and not delayed until after the appetite has passed away (this does not apply to "false appetite" of drunkards and the "munchies" that often follows the intake of marijuana). If the meal is delayed, the stomach will be filled with bad humours.

There is no greater harm than to eat to complete satisfaction after a long period of going without food. This places a great stress upon the digestive powers, and people sometimes die from overeating after a period of true starvation. The damage is not necessarily from overeating, but from the choking of the channels which carry the humoral vapors to the proper areas of the body.

The basic rule for one who wishes to maintain health is: do not eat unless there is a true appetite and unless the stomach and small intestine have been emptied of the preceding meal.

After Eating

A light activity such as walking after a meal allows the food to move into the lower part of the stomach where digestion can be carried on readily, especially if one has a sense of tiredness or desire to lie down. Mental excitement, emotion, and excessive exercise all hinder digestion.

Fruitarian Diet

All of my acquaintances who have experimented with solid-fruit diets for long periods reported rather distressing results, and often serious illness. I wondered about this for quite some time, and was answered by my teacher, the Hakim. He explained that it is not wise to consume "tenuous" things in quantity or to make them the basis of a meal, because they are very quickly assimilated into the body and thus overoxidize the blood. This surely would explain the prevalence of hepatitis among fruitarians, as this is an affliction of the liver, which would have too much superfluous by-products to deal with.

How Much to Eat?

The standard size of a meal depends on general condition and activity of the person. A normally healthy person should eat enough without producing a feeling of heaviness, or a sense of tightness of the solar plexus area. After eating, there should be no rumbling of the stomach, or sloshing of the food on movement. Nausea, taste of the food in belches, and lingering of taste of the meal are all signs that the meal was too heavy. A properly moderate meal will be shown by a moderate pulse and ability to breathe fully. Sometimes, as when one is ill, a full meal cannot be properly taken at one sitting. In such a case, the number of things eaten should be increased, but their quantities reduced.

Foods that are easily and quickly digested should not be taken simultaneously with foods which are slowly digested. The food that is digested first will, being lighter, float over the other food, trapping it. Unable to enter the blood, it will be retained unnecessarily long in the stomach and begin fermenting, resulting in gas and belching.

Liquids with Food

All liquids taken in simultaneously with food dilute the gastric juices and are therefore not recommended with meals. Nor should much liquid be taken directly after a meal, for it causes the food to leave the lining of the stomach and float about. If there is a very great thirst just after a meal, it is best to satisfy it with cold water—the colder it is, the less will be needed to quench the thirst. When the initial process of digestion is over—evidenced by a feeling of lightness in the upper part of the diaphragm—some tea may be taken, preferably one that aids digestion, such as peppermint.

Incompatibilities between Foods

There are simple rules for combining foods according to their compatibility. In India it is always stressed that milk should not

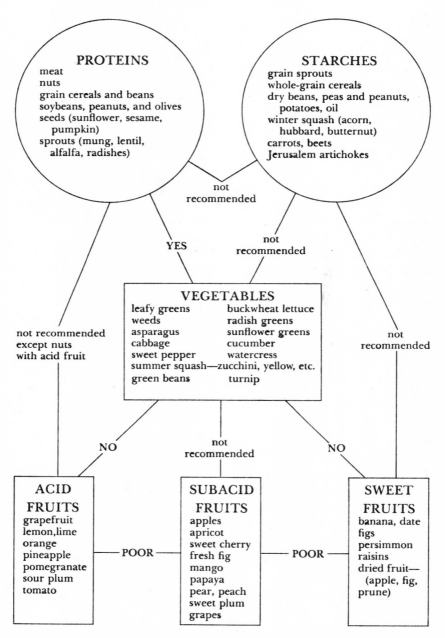

Avocados are best combined with acid or subacid fruits or green vegetables. All melons should be eaten alone. *Do not mix* more than four foods from any one classification. At one meal, *do not mix* food from more than two classifications.

be taken with sour (cold) foods; fish should not be taken with milk; meat should not be cooked over live coals. The chart gives basic guidelines to follow in combining foods.

About Meat Eating

Many intelligent people are questioning the consumption of meat in our culture. The first reason to avoid meat from the commercial food-processing industry is that most animals have been injected with various hormones and chemicals that accelerate or otherwise alter their growth cycles. Mass-raised chickens are usually forced to mature within seven weeks, and are stimulated with chemicals and electric lights twenty-four hours per day to keep them from resting.

The slaughtering methods of the cattle industry are particularly inhumane and, in addition to being "fattened up" with the help of injections, cattle experience extreme fear at the time of death (as they can smell the blood and sense the terror and death of their recently killed kin), which triggers the release of toxins into their bodies that are retained in the meat.

Meat is not prohibited by most religious commandments, and I have seen people who do consume meat to be perfectly acceptable as compassionate and sensitive human beings. My own standards require that any meat which I or my family consume must have been grown on totally organic grains, without being forced to maturity, and slaughtered in as humane and compassionate a manner as possible—by calling on the name of God at the time of killing, and leaving the spinal cord intact to prevent release of toxins into the animal's endocrine system. The attitude in which any food is taken from the Earth, be it plant or animal life, contributes to its final vibration, and that vibration is transferred directly to the one who consumes that life. The recipes in this book are intended for kosher or organic meat items, and there are enough farms, communes, and other sources of organically raised meat and poultry in the United States to make them feasible. As a source of protein, "pure" meat need only be consumed once or twice a week; vegetable protein is just as healthful to the body.

If you are unaccustomed to metabolizing large amounts of vegetable protein, you may have to use some protein supplements during a changeover period. An excellent book on vegetarian nutrition and cooking, written in a sensitive style, is *Laurel's Kitchen* (Berkeley: Nilgiri Press, 1977).

Temperature-Balanced Recipes

The following are several dishes constructed according to the principles of humoral or temperature-balanced diet.[1] I have found them to be quite satisfying and delicious. The recipe for bread is especially recommended, as it is quick to make and contains very little sugar or salt.

AFGHAN NAUN BREAD

This bread is traditionally made with a fermented starter, and although dry yeast is used for the necessary leavening, the flavor will not be quite the same without it. Baking in the pit oven also may impart a little flavor which won't be present in oven baking. In spite of all this, however, this should be an acceptable product.

Combine in a medium or large bowl:

  1 package of dry yeast (1 T.)
  1 t. sugar
  ¼ c. lukewarm water

Mix to dissolve yeast and sugar and set aside.

Sift together:

  3 c. sifted whole-wheat flour
  ½ t. salt

and add to yeast mixture.

Measure and add gradually to the flour-yeast mixture

  ¾ c. cold water

---

[1] Recipes adapted from Doris McKellar, *Afghan Cookery* (Kabul: Afghan Book Publishers, 1972), with additional practical advice from Karima Ibrahimkhail and Enayatullah Shahrani.

Mix with the hand as the water is added, adding a bit more if needed to produce a smooth, firm dough—essentially the same consistency as ordinary bread dough. Allow to stand, covered, in a moderately warm place for one hour. The dough will not double in bulk, but drawing a finger across the surface will show small bubbles being formed.

This is about enough dough for one large naun, but for the method of baking required, it is probably better to make two small ones instead.

Preheat the oven to 500° F. and in it preheat a large cookie sheet which has been covered with heavy aluminum foil. Divide the dough into two balls, allow to stand for 5 minutes, and then begin to shape into oval, flat pieces of desired thickness. For regular naun, the pieces will be about 7 by 12 inches and ⅛ to ½ inch thick. The two pieces of regular naun will fit on one cookie sheet. After the regular naun is shaped, dip three fingers in cold water and make three lengthwise grooves down the center of each.

Place the shaped naun on the hot cookie sheet and bake immediately until the dough is set and just beginning to brown—6 minutes, probably. If the bread has not browned sufficiently, turn on the broiler to complete browning. Remove from oven and serve warm or cold, cut in 4-inch squares. An electric skillet or heavy griddle, ungreased, can also be used quite satisfactorily for baking naun. Size of naun, time, and temperature would have to be adjusted for each situation.

Naun is served without butter or any fat added, is often used to pick up other foods, and is particularly important in the eating of soup.

VETCH SOUP

Soak overnight in cold water:

½ c. dried mung beans
½ c. dried red beans

Place in a large kettle or pressure cooker and cook until soft:

½ c. dried vetch (substitute green split peas if not available)
¼ c. short-grain rice
mung beans and red beans that have been soaked
1 t. salt
4 c. water, including soaking water

Mix and form into balls ½ inch in diameter (vegetarians may omit):

½ lb. ground beef (kosher or organically grown *only*)
¼ t. salt
½ t. red pepper
½ t. black pepper

Heat in saucepan:

¼ c. vegetable fat

Add and brown lightly:

1 medium onion, diced fine

Remove from fire, cool slightly.

Add and then cook until all water is evaporated:

2 c. water
¼ c. tomato, fresh or canned
meat balls (if used)

Add to this mixture the following, and heat gently:

all cooked grains and beans
1 c. yogurt or sour cream
1 t. to 1 T. powdered dill
1 t. to 2 t. salt, to taste

Serve hot in individual soup plates.

Serves 4–6

AUSHAK
(Ravioli with leek filling)

Place in a bowl and mix:

3 c. sifted white flour
1 t. salt

Add:

⅞ c. cold water

Stir to form a very stiff dough. Divide dough into 3 balls, cover, and set aside.

Wash:

1 bundle of leeks or green onions

Cut into ¼-inch pieces and wash again. Squeeze with hand to remove water. Place in a bowl:

2–3 c. chopped leeks
1 t. salt
¼ t. red pepper

Mix and squeeze to remove more water.

Add:

1 T. vegetable oil, set aside

Drain about 1 qt. yogurt to yield 2 cups. Place in bowl and mix:

2 c. drained yogurt
3 cloves fresh garlic, ground, or ¼ t. dried
1 t. salt

Set aside.

To prepare kosher meat sauce, heat in a saucepan:

½ c. vegetable oil

Add and brown:

1 medium onion, chopped

Add:

1 lb. ground beef, crumbled
½ t. salt
1 t. black pepper

Brown the meat. Then add:

½ c. tomato juice
2 c. water

Boil until liquid evaporates and sauce is oily.

To prepare dough: Roll out one ball of dough on a floured board until it is very thin ($\frac{1}{16}$th inch). Cut with a round cutter (1½ to 2 inches in diameter) or in squares the same size. Put a few of the drained leeks on half of the dough, moisten edges, and seal shut tightly. They should not open during the cooking. Place on tray or cookie sheet and cover until all are prepared, repeating this process with the remaining dough and leeks.

Heat in a kettle:

2 qts. water

Drop several ravioli in at a time, using a little cold water to keep from boiling over. Boil for 10 minutes. Place ½ of the yogurt on a serving platter. Lift the cooked ravioli with slotted spoon, arrange over the yogurt. Cover with remaining yogurt and sprinkle with:

1 T. pulverized dry mint

Top with the remaining meat sauce and serve at once.

Serves 6–8

QABALI PAULOW
(Rice with Carrots and Raisins)

This is probably the most widely known and popular of the many paulows.

Heat in a kettle or pressure cooker:

½ c. vegetable oil

Dice and add to oil, sauté until brown:

1 med. onion

Add and brown lightly:

1 lb. kosher or organically grown chicken, lamb, or beef

Add:

2 c. water
1 t. salt
1 to 1½ t. mixed spices (equal parts of cinnamon, cloves, cumin, and cardamom) ground

Cover and simmer, or cook under pressure, until the meat is tender. Remove the meat from the juice and set aside. This juice will be used for cooking the rice.

Wash and scrape or peel:

2 medium carrots

Cut into toothpick-sized pieces.

Heat in a small saucepan:

¼ c. vegetable oil

Add:

1 t. honey
sliced carrots

Cook until carrots are lightly browned. If carrots are too tough, add:

½ c. water

Simmer until tender and water has evaporated. Remove carrots from oil and add to the oil:

1 c. dark seedless raisins

Cook until the raisins begin to swell. Remove and set aside with the carrots. If almonds are used, they should also be lightly browned in the oil and set aside. Save the oil for the rice.

Optional additions:

¼ t. saffron
2 T. blanched almonds
2 T. blanched pistachios, crushed or whole

To cook the rice, begin by boiling the kosher meat juices and add:

2 c. long-grain rice
1½ t. salt
boiling water sufficient to bring level of liquid 2 inches above the rice

Cook until all water is absorbed and rice is tender. Test for doneness by removing one grain and squeezing between thumb and finger. Then, when done, add to the cooked rice:

the reserved oil in which carrots were cooked
saffron (optional)

Mix gently through the rice. Then, to complete cooking and blend flavors, put kosher meat and rice in a large casserole, cover, and set in a 300°F. oven for 20–30 minutes. To serve, place the kosher meat in the center of a large platter. Mound the rice over the top and sprinkle with carrots, raisins, almonds, and pistachios, if these are used.

Serves 6–8

CHALOW
(White Rice)

Combine:

3 c. long-grain white rice
1 t. salt
2 qts. boiling water

Cook until rice is tender. Strain and place rice in an ovenware dish.

Mix separately:

¼ c. vegetable oil
½ c. water
½ t. salt

Pour this mixture over the drained rice and toss gently with pancake turner or large rice server until oil coats all rice. Cover and place in 300°F. oven for 20 to 30 minutes to complete cooking.

To serve: Mound rice on a large platter. If desired, pour over the rice an additional:

¼ c. vegetable oil or melted butter

Accompany with a vegetable sauce such as Saulan.

Serves 6–8

SAULAN
(Vegetable Sauce)

Cut into 1-inch cubes:

1½ lb. vegetables of choice (cauliflower, cabbage, or spinach) (fresh peas or fresh green beans) (eggplant or summer squash)

Heat in kettle:

¾ c. vegetable oil

Add and brown lightly:

cubed vegetables
2 medium onions, sliced
2 cloves garlic, minced

Add:

1½ t. salt
¼ t. black pepper
½ t. red pepper

Cook slowly until vegetables are browned lightly. Then, to complete the cooking of the vegetable, add to sauce and simmer 5 to 10 minutes:

½ c. water

Serve as a sauce over the Chalow.

Serves 8

BURAUNEE BAUNJAUN
(Fried Eggplant with Yogurt)

Combine and mix well:

1 c. drained yogurt, drained at least one hour
3 cloves fresh garlic, minced, or 1 t. dried
1 t. salt

Set aside. This mixture is used in a number of meat and vegetable dishes.

Wash, peel, and slice in ½-inch slices lengthwise:

3 medium eggplants

Score slices lightly with a knife, spread on a board or flat pan, and sprinkle with ¼ t. salt. Allow to stand 10–15 minutes to draw out some of the bitter juices. Wipe dry.

Heat in kettle or frying pan:

1 c. vegetable oil

Fry eggplant slices until light brown, remove, and set aside.

Dice very finely and add to oil:

1 medium onion

Fry until lightly browned.

Add to oil and onion:

eggplant slices
1 t. salt
½ c. tomato sauce or 1 c. tomato juice
¼ t. red pepper
¼ c. chopped green pepper
¼ c. water

Cook slowly until eggplant is tender. To serve: Put half of the yogurt and garlic mixture on a serving platter. Arrange eggplant slices, top with remaining yogurt mixture, and spoon some eggplant sauce over the top. Serve with naun bread.

Serves 4–6

BULANNEE
(Fried Turnovers with Leeks)

Stir together in a mixing bowl:

6 c. sifted white flour
2 t. salt

Add and mix and knead to form a stiff, elastic bread dough:

1¾ to 2 c. water

Cover dough and set aside.

Sort and wash carefully:

1 lb. leeks (or green onion tops)

Cut into ¼-inch pieces (there should be 4 c. after chopping).

Put leeks into a kettle of water and wash again. As they are removed from this water, squeeze with the hands to remove water and place in another bowl. Add to the chopped, drained leeks:

1½ t. salt
½ t. red pepper

Squeeze the leeks with hand until they begin to soften. Add:

1 T. vegetable oil

Mix and set aside.

To prepare dough, divide and shape into balls the size of walnuts. This recipe should yield 18 or 20 of this size. Roll each circle out very thin on a lightly floured board to no more than 1/16th of an inch. The diameter of the circle should be 9 to 10 inches. If these are tough after cooking, it will be because the dough was not rolled out thin enough.

On half of each circle, spread:

3 to 4 T. drained leeks

Moisten the edges of the dough, fold over in half and seal. In a shallow pan heat 1½ c. vegetable oil for frying and fry two turnovers at a time, browning well on both sides. Serve warm. This dish is served on picnics, birthdays, and for other parties.

Serves 6–8

DRIED FRUIT COMPOTE

Wash all of the ingredients and place in one bowl:

4 c. dried apricots
4 c. dark seedless raisins
2 c. light raisins

Cover with cold water to 2 inches above the fruit. Cover and refrigerate for two days.

In a second bowl place:

2 c. English or California walnuts (Persian walnuts)
2 c. pistachio nuts
2 c. dried apricot seeds or almonds

Add water the same as above, cover and set aside.

As the skins soften on the nuts, they should all be peeled. After the two days of soaking, combine:

apricots, raisins
peeled nuts
1 c. drained maraschino cherries, halved

To serve: Spoon fruit and nuts into individual dessert dishes or cups, being sure that some of the cherries and nuts are in each cup for garnish. The juice is served with the fruit, with ½ inch to 1 inch of juice in each serving.

Recommended Readings

Beiler, Henry. *Food Is Your Best Medicine.* London: Neville Spearman, 1968.

Chen, Philip S. *Chemistry: Inorganic, Organic, and Biological.* New York: Barnes & Noble, 1968.

Fogarty International Center. *A Barefoot Doctor's Manual (The American Translation of the Official Chinese Paramedical Manual).* Philadelphia: Running Press, 1977.

Heritage, Ford. *Composition and Facts about Food.* Mokelumne Hill, Calif.: Health Research, 1971.

Lee Foundation for Nutritional Research, *Portfolio of Reprints for the Doctor.* Milwaukee: Lee Foundation for Nutritional Research, 1974.

Robertson, Laurel, Carol Flinders, and Bronwen Godfrey. *Laurel's Kitchen: A Handbook for Vegetarian Cookery and Nutrition.* Berkeley: Nilgiri Press, 1977.

Chapter 5

Detoxification: the Modified Fast

The axiom "Fasting is the best medicine" was given in Chapter 2 as one of the most important principles of natural medicine. Unfortunately, in the past decades, as the natural-foods trends grew, many people have been very forward in pressing their ideas upon others. This has caused many people to be "turned off" to otherwise sound principles. The idea of fasting, great and necessary as it is, is perhaps the greatest area of wrong thinking among the general public. "How can we live eating *nothing*?" they may ask. This may sound absurd until one looks more closely at the matter.

If an automobile develops a sudden clanking in the engine as it is being propelled down the road at sixty miles per hour, you would not think of suggesting that a passenger climb out on the hood and check the engine. Or one would not begin repairs of any real mechanical problem with the motor running. Fasting is applying this same logic to the body. When one realizes that all illness *originates* in wrong dietary habits and that the body itself is the only mechanism capable of effecting a true, complete cure, then the processes going on in restoring health can be understood.

If the dietary habits of those who became sick were examined, one would see that there was something—or many things—in their habits that could be considered quite bizarre. A man's wife died of cancer of the brain, but her husband was very adamant that she had eaten only the "best" foods. Even allowing for the toxins inherent in even the best supermarket foods today, I was puzzled at this apparent cruel blow of fate. After a while, this man did confess that the only thing strange about his wife's diet was that she had eaten a heaping bowl of buttered popcorn every night of her life for the past twenty years!

Another woman who died of cancer was reported by her husband to have had some peculiar hungers—like eating sandwiches composed solely of white bread and horseradish; the woman was frequently seen weeping at the dinner table from the pungency of the horseradish. Another woman remarked that her five-year-old daughter (who had asthma) was always insisting that she put garlic on everything. The mother was about to call in a psychiatrist when the girl asked for garlic on ice cream.

What strikes me about this case is that the girl's body *knew* what was needed—garlic is one of the most effective blood purifiers and phlegm-reducers. So, the procedure to follow is to understand that the body always knows how and has the capacity to heal itself; by knowing this, one can assist nature in this most remarkable phenomenon.

The theory underlying fasting is that the body possesses a competent mechanism for eliminating the by-products of poor nutrition as well as the toxic effects of worry, grief, and anger, which often have more to do with onset of illness than any other factors.

Let us recall the statements of Dr. Mayo and the West Coast natural physician who never saw a healthy colon. The latter once commented wisely, "Death begins in the colon." The feces are the natural expulsion of by-products of normal systemic digestion, and there are normal limits to this process.

The normal evacuation time depends somewhat on the type of food consumed but, in general, most foods should be thoroughly digested and passed out of the body within twelve to twenty-four hours. For those who go for two or three—or more—days without a movement, there is without doubt an illness being made. And, if proper elimination is not attained, illness will result. Yes, it is true that some people go through life constipated, but we are not interested in mere survival but in establishing a fully functioning harmonious life organism. The person who *is* able to "survive" on poor diet and elimination still pays a great toll in such ailments as headache, nervousness, gall-bladder trouble, constipation, and so on.

It is not only *no* elimination that can indicate trouble to come; examination of the stool can quickly point up a faulty elimination. Most Americans are so fastidious that they would never want to see their own by-products. In the East, people squat down and defecate in a way that allows them to examine their own waste. This is not meant to be distasteful or a joke, but only that one should be able to engage in this kind of examination without feeling in danger of contracting disease from such "untouchable" matters.

The Healthy Stool

The normal healthy stool should be (1) held together, (2) watery and solid parts equally mixed throughout, (3) soft and like honey in consistency, (4) easily expelled, (5) of a color tending to yellow (if it is the color of the food eaten: i.e., if green after broccoli, digestion has been incomplete), (6) not entirely odorless, but not of a noxious odor, (7) emitted without sound of gurgling, foaming, or flatulence, (8) passed at times proper for a healthy person, and (9) of a bulk nearly the same as that of the food eaten.

If one or several of these characteristics are absent from one's bowel movements, it is a sign that the digestive process is off somewhere in the system. The lower bowel or colon is the counterpart to a drain in a sink. If a drain pipe becomes clogged, one does not imagine that pouring more water and refuse into the sink would help the problem.

Fasting in human beings is the same thing as turning off the water in a clogged sink. The body has the capacity to eliminate accumulated toxic materials and superfluous matter, but it cannot do so while a constant barrage of excess and poor food is being poured into it. So, the first step is to cut off the water— in this case, food. Contrary to what many people think and recommend, total abstinence from food is not the only way to fast. Total abstinence is a radical method for those who are physically and mentally prepared to take it up. But it is not for every one. One who fasts entirely for one day a week will generally be in much better health than one who fasts a week a year. The body, as a natural mechanism, strives for balance, and once per week is more balanced than once a year. So many books purport to give a "big-bang" resolution to health problems, yet it is rather by regular, controlled living that true health will be gained.

The Nutritional Profile

One of the problems with therapeutic diets and programs is that they include recommendations for what is required by the *healthy* or normal body. Yet this is a rare specimen in our culture. What is needed is to determine what is going on inside your own body, at the present time.

If one wants to get some idea of how well or poorly his or her own body is functioning, the Nutritional Profile developed by R. J. Baumann will give a clear picture, is quick and easy to do, and is a first step in taking over responsibility for one's own health. With the Nutritional Profile, we learn something about several processes of the body: temperature, pulse rate, and acidity of the saliva and urine. The Nutritional Profile can be done by each person individually, and does not require any expensive equipment.

Temperature

If it is recalled that the body is in many ways like a nuclear reactor in that there is an inner source of heat—in this case, the metabolism of food—we can learn most readily from the temperature just how efficiently this inner mechanism is working. The normal temperature of the adult body is usually given as 98.6 degrees Fahrenheit, taken orally, and somewhat higher rectally. Lower or higher temperatures usually represent some malfunction of the bodily system, although from the temperature alone it is difficult if not impossible to determine what is wrong. We know, though, that a temperature of 95 degrees would be a fatal condition, because life is not sustained for long at this temperature. On the other hand, a temperature of 107 degrees will also cause death. So it is within this relatively restricted range of some twelve or so degrees that life carries on its activities. If one took a temperature consistently low, say around 97.0 degrees, it would mean that combustion of the nutrients was being carried on inefficiently. Just as a lowered current flowing through an electrical line will result in lowered illumination in a light bulb, resulting in strained vision, a lowered temperature in time will cause a great deal of excessive work for the body to properly carry on the work of full and complete digestion. The organs that must pitch in to help the digestion themselves become worn down, and eventually an entire organ is damaged. A consistently raised temperature means that there is something overheating the system, and an overabundance of heat always results in burnout and damage of one kind or another. Actually, the normal temperature of a truly healthy person would be more in the range of 99.0 degrees Fahrenheit. The temperature should fluctuate during different times of day. For example, the low temperature is reached around 4 A.M., after a night of sleep with no food intake. The heat can be turned down, so to speak, since the major work is finished. The temperature will rise from noon to 2 P.M., because the body is fully geared up and operating at maximum efficiency. This is why it is recommended to eat meat (if one does) at the noon meal, when the body is most able to assimilate it properly.

Pulse

The normal pulse in an adult is 70 beats per minute for men, and slightly more for women. If one has a very low pulse, say 50 to 55, it may mean that the body is entirely clogged with matter that cannot be eliminated. If the body is extremely toxic, the pulse may soar to 90 or 100 in a wild effort to eliminate the toxins, which are literally poisoning the system. During a healing crisis, the temperature and pulse will both rise, which shows a coordinated effort of the body to speed the blood through the body, with raised heat of combustion, to clean out the system. The great error made in treating disease by conventional medical means is that a fever is usually suppressed, when it is by this very means that the body is trying to restore health!

There is a great deal to learn about pulse. The healers of China, Afghanistan, India, Iran, and many other nations are competent in what is called "pulse diagnosis." This is a method of measuring not just the *number* of times the pulse crosses the measuring point, but also its various qualities: the depth of the vessel carrying the blood, expansion and contraction of the pulse, strong or weak beating, the time between beats of the pulse, cycles of distance between pulse beats, the moisture content on the skin above the pulse, and several other factors. This component method of measuring the pulse gives the healer an exact idea of what is transpiring within that specific person's body, rather than a simple recording of a norm. I myself have on at least three occasions had a healer give *me* the specific symptoms of illness, and one threw in a description of my cultural and geographical background for good measure!

Saliva pH

This is nothing more than recording the relative acidity or alkalinity of the fluid of the mouth. It must be measured at least half an hour after consumption of any food or drink, so that these substances will not alter the reading.

The normal pH range of the mouth is 6.5 to 7.5. One can determine the pH of one's own saliva by buying a roll of Nitrazine tape, which is available at practically any drugstore. A small piece is torn off, wet with the saliva, and then read from a color-coded chart on the package.

It is best to measure the reading several times during the day, at the same time that the temperature and pulse are recorded. This will allow one to see if there are any patterns in relation to the foods consumed and also serve as a personalized record of the processes within one's own system.

Urine pH

The acid-alkaline range of the urine is measured in a similar manner to the saliva. The normal pH range of the urine is lower, or more acid, because the end product of elimination is always acid. Thus, if one had a saliva reading of 4.5, it would mean that there was excessive acidity in the mouth and a sign that some backup in the system was occurring. In other words, the value of the saliva was reversed and had the value of urine. The pH value of the urine is 5.5 to 6.5, and if it measures consistently low (in the 4.0 to 4.5 range) it would mean that the elimination was overtaxed and constantly emitting acid-toxic matter, when it should recover to the normal range after eliminating the by-products of digestion. The chart on page 72, with spaces for recording all of these four factors, will quickly give a simple yet accurate picture of what is happening with four very important functions of the body. If one's saliva pH is too acid, it means that digestion (which really begins in the mouth) is off from the *beginning*.

The Detoxification Program

It is clear that the majority of American adults need some kind of detoxification regimen to cleanse the body of accumulated mucus and toxic materials. If one makes a Nutritional Profile and finds the temperature and pulse low, and acid saliva and urine (and there are no other symptoms), it is likely that a detoxification program is in order.

The means to accomplish this is quite simple, but does require willpower and concentration. The first step is to construct one's own Nutritional Profile for at least two days before undertaking the regimen. This will give an indication of what is going on in the body and provides some statistics to measure against those for the period of detoxification.

It is possible to conduct a detoxification on a modified fast at any time, but for those who have never done it before, it may be wise to set aside three or more days to concentrate exclusively upon the program, so that there is less risk of abandoning it if something interferes.

The following is called a "modified" fast, because a considerable range of foods may be eaten. However, there are some foods which are prohibited. These are all fruits; all condiments;

all sugars in any form, even honey; all coffee, wine, liquor, cigarettes, drugs, or any other stimulant. In place of these, the intake of fresh green vegetables is increased. The detoxification foods list on page 73 gives the foods that can be consumed.

NUTRITIONAL PROFILE

Name

Week of

		Tem-perature	Pulse	Urine pH	Saliva pH
Sunday	Wake-up				
	2 P.M.				
	8 P.M.				
Monday	Wake-up				
	2 P.M.				
	8 P.M.				
Tuesday	Wake-up				
	2 P.M.				
	8 P.M.				
Wednesday	Wake-up				
	2 P.M.				
	8 P.M.				
Thursday	Wake-up				
	2 P.M.				
	8 P.M.				
Friday	Wake-up				
	2 P.M.				
	8 P.M.				
Saturday	Wake-up				
	2 P.M.				
	8 P.M.				

Notes

While no specific amount is specified, it is intended that each person eat only a normal portion at each mealtime. Salads can be consumed freely, and since oil and vinegar as well as other ingredients for salad dressing are prohibited, it is good to make a rich and delicious dressing from fresh yogurt and herbs. Vegetables, if cooked, should be steamed lightly for no more than five to seven minutes.

Eat *only* the foods on the following list:

DETOXIFICATION FOODS LIST

Vegetables: asparagus, beet, broccoli, Brussels sprouts, carrot, celery, chard (Swiss), cucumber, eggplant, endive, garlic, kohlrabi, lettuce (leaf), mushrooms, mustard greens, onion, parsley, parsnip, pepper (green, hot), potato (white), radish, spinach, squash (zucchini), tomato, watercress

Legumes: beans (green, snap), peas

Grains and flours: wheat germ, bran, oatmeal

Fruits: papaya, avocado

Seeds: pumpkin, squash, sesame, sunflower

Nuts: Brazil nut (for protein), piñon

Meats: chicken (white meat), lamb, turkey

Fish: bass, trout, perch

Dairy products: butter, yogurt

Herbs: chives, sweet basil, dill

Beverages: green herb teas only

Special Instructions: Coffee or chickory-root enemas at wake-up

During a state of detoxification, there is much elimination of **excess** matters from the body, and much of this must pass out through the kidneys, spleen and other organs, especially to the colon. To assist this process, which is entirely natural, it is recommended to take at least one enema per day.

The Coffee Enema

Absurd as this idea may sound, it was developed by one of the leading nontoxic therapists in the world, Max Gerson, M.D. He was working to develop a cure for a rare type of tuberculosis called lupus vulgaris. After much research and verification of results, he announced that he had indeed found the cure for this disease and that this therapy (which also included a detoxification program similar to the one given above) cured not only lupus tuberculosis but a whole range of other chronic and degenerative diseases, including emphysema, colitis, stomach ulcer, cancer, and others. He was laughed out of his profession and expelled from the American Medical Association. Gerson was a medical doctor who had learned in his native Vienna that the simple methods of nature's curative mechanisms produced the only real cures, and that all other efforts were merely palliative—that is, they only masked symptoms that were sure to reappear sooner or later.

Even though Dr. Gerson was called a medical genius by Albert Schweitzer, he was hounded by his profession and the law, and died in disgrace. His entire therapy is available in his book *A Cancer Therapy*, written in a totally scientific and professional vocabulary, for those trained in scientific methods who may be skeptics. His daughter has carried on her father's treatment, and the coffee enema has become a regular feature of most of the drugless therapies in the Western hemisphere.

The reason the coffee enema works is that the caffeine is readily absorbed into the lining of the colon, and it also travels up the hemorrhoidal portal vein, to stimulate the gall bladder and spleen, causing them to "dump" their contents so that the eliminative process can proceed quickly, without damaging these organs.

There are so many people who have benefited from this alone—without any herbs or other remedies—that it does not need proof here. There are many M.D.s in the United States who use it, as well as hundreds of naturopaths and chiropractors who do nutritional detoxification. One of the most respected naturopaths in the Southwest even offers coffee colonics, which irrigate the entire colon with coffee. It has been successful in aiding the elimination of gross amounts of phlegm during asthma attacks.

If one has a regular bowel movement on waking in the morning and then takes the coffee enema, one can see just how incomplete the elimination is, for additional matter is expelled in an amount nearly equal to the original movement! Especially women who have painful menstruation have found relief by taking coffee enemas for several days prior to onset of flow. Remember, however, that coffee, if used frequently, will lose its diuretic action as the body becomes acclimated to it. In addition, it is not recommended to take coffee enemas at night, as sleeplessness may result.

Chickory Root for Enemas

The use of chickory root in conditions of the liver, spleen, and kidneys has a long history in traditional medicine. Chickory root is an ingredient (an adulteration) in most coffees sold in the supermarket. When roasted alone, chickory yields from 45 percent to 65 percent extractive matter, while coffee yields only 21 percent to 25 percent. When added to coffee, chickory gives a bitter taste and the dark, rich color, and serves to correct the stimulating effect of caffeine. It is more suitable than coffee for people who suffer chronic biliousness and constipation. A decoction of one ounce of the root to a pint of water has been found effective in jaundice, liver enlargements, gout, and rheumatic complaints. The leaves may be added occasionally to salads, but the leaves should be blanched to remove their bitterness.

For these reasons, I personally use chickory root rather than coffee enemas for general detoxification purposes. (In addition, with the cost of coffee so high today, it is more economical.)

Prepare a one-pint decoction of chickory root, or use the directions given for coffee in the next section.

Chickory root is employed in many of the preparations in

the Formulary, and should always be on hand in the home herbal inventory.

The recommended method of administering the enema is given below.

HOW TO ADMINISTER THE ENEMA

Materials Needed:
1. Regular ground drip coffee (not instant), or 1 oz. chickory root.
2. Enema bag, open-pour spout type, with shut-off valve.
3. Distilled, nursery, or spring water (the kind sold in glass bottles only). Do *not* use tap water, as it may contain fluoride which will not boil out.
4. Vaseline (for lubricating tip of nozzle).

Coffee Preparation:
1. Place two tablespoons of coffee or chickory root in one pint of distilled water. Boil for five minutes. Allow to stand until body temperature. (A regular coffee percolator or a coffee machine may be used to brew the coffee.)
2. If you are to take more than one enema per day, you may make up an extra amount, and keep refrigerated until time for use. Use a sealed jar, and reheat to body temperature before using.

Taking the Enema:
1. Hang enema bag not higher than 24 inches above the body entrance of hose tip.
2. Pour one pint of liquid, at body temperature, into enema bag.
3. Lubricate nozzle tip with Vaseline.
4. Place towel or newspaper around area of buttocks in case of accidental spillage from hose or premature expulsion.
5. *Lie on right side* and gently insert hose tip into anal opening.
6. Release hose valve. Liquid will flow into colon. If too much pressure is felt, close valve until pressure stops, then release valve and continue.
7. When enema bag is emptied of contents, close valve and remove nozzle tip.
8. Retain fluid ten to fifteen minutes (but not longer than fifteen), then evacuate.

This detoxification program is not dangerous to adults, although one should have a physical examination by a competent health practitioner before commencing it. It is recommended that administration to children be done only with supervision by a physician.

The effects of the detoxification should be evident within one day by a lowering of the saliva pH, meaning that the backup of toxins is receding and normal enzyme function is occurring in the mouth at the first stage of digestion. After three days, a definite improvement in the sense of well-being should be apparent, with the temperature and pulse becoming more normal.

It may be that after years and years of dietary indiscretion, results are not so rapid. It is not possible to achieve instantaneous results with any natural modality, for the body does not work in an instant. It will take time to recover full functioning of organs, as the body rebuilds damaged tissue. It is most important to record what one feels during a detoxification and note any gross or subtle changes. We often can find the clue to imbalance in the food we eat with no more than this kind of simple procedure.

There is no need to make any special changeover diet after this program, but in general we should strive to consume the basic recommended foods in greater quantities.

It is well to remember our animal friends, dogs and cats, who, on their own, refuse to eat during times of illness. Since we are constantly in a process of trying to build health, it will prove of greatest benefit to follow a regular schedule of allowing the body a chance to eliminate excess waste and toxins by detoxifying.

Recommended Readings

There are a great many books today on fasting. Some of them are clearly full of misinformation, and can be considered dangerous. Those on this list are in keeping with the true principles of natural medicine, and, while they are not the only ones, they are accurate and safe to use, if followed properly.

Al-Ghazzali. *The Mysteries of Fasting*. Lahore: Ashraf Press, 1968.

Bragg, Paul. *The Miracle of Fasting*. Santa Ana, Calif.: Health Science, n.d.

Ehret, Arnold. *Mucusless Diet Healing System*. Beaumont, Calif.: Ehret Publishing Company, 1922.

Gerson, Max, M.D. *A Cancer Therapy*, 2d ed. Del Mar, Calif.: Totality Books, 1975.

Walker, N. W. *Raw Vegetable Juices*. New York: Pyramid Books, 1970.

Part Two
The Formulary

Tables of Weights and Measures

TABLE 1: LIQUID MEASURES

U.S.

1 tablespoon	= 3 teaspoons	
1 ounce	= 2 tablespoons	= 0.03 liters
1 gill	= 4 fluid ounces	= 0.12 liters
1 cup	= 8 fluid ounces	= 0.24 liters
1 pint	= 2 cups	= 0.48 liters
1 quart	= 2 pints	= 0.96 liters
1 gallon	= 4 quarts	= 3.78 liters

Metric

1 centiliter	= 10 mililiters	= 0.34 fluid ounces
1 deciliter	= 10 centiliters	= 3.38 fluid ounces
1 liter	= 10 deciliters	= 1.06 quarts
1 decaliter	= 10 liters	= 2.64 gallons

Apothecary

1 minim	= 0.06 mililiters	
1 fluid dram	= 60 minims	= 3.70 mililiters

TABLE 2: DRY MEASURES

Avoirdupois

---

1 grain	=	0.06 grams	
1 dram	= 27.3 grains	=	1.77 grams
1 ounce	= 16 drams	=	28.35 grams
1 pound	= 16 ounces	=	4.53 grams

Apothecary (Troy)

---

1 scruple	= 20 grains	=	1.30 grams
1 dram	= 3 scruples	=	3.89 grams
1 ounce	= 8 drams	=	37.10 grams
1 pound	= 12 ounces	=	3.73 grams

Metric

---

1 centigram	= 10 miligrams	=	0.15 grains
1 decigram	= 10 centigrams	=	1.54 grains
1 gram	= 10 decigrams	=	15.43 grains
1 decagram	= 10 grams	=	0.35 ounces
1 hectogram	= 10 decagrams	=	3.53 ounces
1 kilogram	= 10 hectograms	=	2.20 pounds

TABLE 3: APPROXIMATE EQUIVALENTS BETWEEN THE APOTHECARY AND METRIC SYSTEMS

Apothecaries		*Metric*
1/60th grain	=	1 mg.
1 grain	=	60 mg.
15 grains	=	1 gm.
15 or 16 minims	=	1 cc.
1 dram	=	4 cc. or gm.
1 ounce	=	30 cc. or gm.
1 pint	=	475 or 500 cc.

TABLE 4: HOUSEHOLD MEASURES

For the preparation of solutions used externally, for the administration of certain drugs where great accuracy is not essential, and for the emergency preparation of solutions where accurate weighing and measuring apparatus is not available (such as treatment in the home), it is often very convenient to know the capacities of various common household containers:

Household	Apothecary	Metric
Less than a teaspoon	= a few grains	
Teaspoon	= 1 dram	= 4 cc.
Dessert spoon	= 2 drams	= 8 cc.
Tablespoon	= 4 drams	= 15 cc.
Cup	= 7 ounces	= 200 cc.
Tumbler	= 8 ounces	= 250 cc.
Fruit jar	= ½ pt., 1 pt.	= 250, 500
	1 qt., ½ gal.	= 1000, 2000 cc.

Using the Formulary

1. Once you have a good general idea of where and what the signs are, look up the section heading ("Head," "Stomach," etc.) for the part affected. The general descriptions of signs are fairly complete, so if you do not find the signs you need in the section headings, refer to the index for a more thorough listing of signs.

2. Each section gives a general explanation of the humoral imbalance, i.e., whether the blood, phlegm, or yellow or black bile humour is out of harmony. You will sometimes find instructions with specific ingredients for making the preparation to correct this imbalance. At other times, a general directive is given, such as "purge the phlegm." In these cases, you must refer to the descriptions of single and compound remedies for the humours, which are given in the following pages. After these general directions are followed, a suggestion is given for dietary regimen, massage, local application to relieve any swellings, itching, and inflammations.

3. In making the herbal preparations, general herbal apothecary language is employed: "Make a decoction, salve, oxymel," and so forth. To prepare these remedies, follow instructions given in the general directions for compounding herbs in the following pages.

4. It is especially recommended that before applying a remedy, or attempting to, the entire section preceding the specific sections be read, so you have an overall idea of the range of application of the remedies and other suggestions for restoring the body to optimum health.

Nature's Healing Herbs

For those who have experience in using the harmless herbs of bodily correction, there is no need to justify their use. The plant kingdom provides the raw materials for many of today's allopathic remedies, and, as recently as 1926, one of the leading reference works for medical doctors included many herbal recommendations.

Our knowledge of the use of herbs goes back to earliest recorded history, some 4500 years ago, and anthropological data reveal sustained use of herbs by man over nearly three million years.

In selecting the herbs for inclusion in this volume, it was recognized that there are many thousands of herbs which are used throughout the world. While there is no doubt that most if not all of these have value, we have included only those which have found a sustained use in the traditions of herbal practice. It would serve no useful purpose here to present all herbs and their many applications. Often the herbs recommended in one part of the world are less effective when processed for shipment to other lands, and many of them are simply unavailable in the United States.

The method employed in listing herbs in this volume is to give the proper formula for a specific *set of signs*. While many comprehensive volumes are available which give full botanical information on herbs, there is still no source for applying them for a specific ailment. The formulas given here are those used by the traditional healers of the East and West and whose use in herbal pharmacopoeia has been established for more than a thousand years.

These formulas have been gathered from several important Persian texts on natural medicine, and appear for the first time in the West in this book. In some cases, substitutions have been made for herbs not available in the United States, or where an herb has gained a reputation for treating a similar ailment in a specific locale. For more specific information on these herbs, the reader is referred to *Indian Herbalogy of North America* by Alma Hutchens (Windsor, Ontario: MERCO, 1974), and *A Modern Herbal* by M. Grieve, Vols. I and II (New York: Dover, 1971).

There are many other herbals of fine quality and complete listings. These are among the best, and are given for ready reference. The bibliography gives a more extended listing.

Obtaining Herbs

The best way of procuring herbs is to grow them and cut them fresh for use or dry them under proper conditions. A surprising number of herbs can easily be grown indoors or out and, with a little morning sunlight, will do quite well. For those who live in rural areas, many "weeds" will prove on close examination to be herbs of value in healing. It is unwise to ingest any plant unless you know for certain what it is, even in small doses. If in doubt, consult a physician who deals with herbs or other expert advisors.

With the growing interest in medicinal herbs today, most health food stores carry fairly complete lines of dried herbs. These can usually be used with safety, although there was a recent case in Arizona in which two children died as a result of ingesting an extremely toxic plant from Mexico that had been mistakenly supplied in place of a harmless herb of very similar appearance. Nature is sometimes very subtle in her differences.

Several firms have recently begun producing herbs prepared in either tablet or capsule form, and these provide a new convenience for herb users. As the use of herbal remedies grows, there will no doubt be a larger product line of such herbs and, since they are prepared under FDA scrutiny, one can rely on their strength and purity.

Each person becomes knowledgeable about herbs, or at least one person within each family, so that expert consultation is available when needed. It is impossible to gain all the desired knowledge of herb use quickly, and thus it is recommended to become familiar with a few herbs at first. Learn how to grow and gather them, what their effects are, and how effective they are for yourself and your family. Remember that herbs are Nature's cure and often take time to work. They work by means of their own "inner knowledge" of the human body and may not have a noticeable effect immediately. Others will produce immediate results. It is important to know what the anticipated effects will be, so that the person to whom they are administered will not become alarmed or disappointed in using them.

The Basic Fifty

One major herb supplier lists more than 800 different herbs in its basic catalogue. This is confusing and frustrating when one is just beginning with herbs, for it is hard to know which are the right or best ones, and some of them are quite expensive and hard to obtain. While on a visit to the West Coast recently, I decided to purchase a supply of those herbs which comprise the basic fifty—those herbs that should be on hand and comprise a beginning inventory for those who wish to use herbs as a regular part of their well-being program. All can be obtained inexpensively at various herbal outlets in this country. Once you have learned about them and realized their benefit, others can be added to this basic list until a complete herbal pharmacopoeia is on hand.

Regardless of how they are packaged when purchased or shipped, they should be stored in airtight glass containers, preferably of an amber hue. There are volatile oils in herbs that react with plastic, thus glass is necessary. Herbs will keep indefinitely if stored properly.

THE BASIC FIFTY

1. Acacia, false	18. Gallnut	35. Plantain,
2. Agrimony	19. Ginger	Common
3. Aloe vera	20. Golden seal	36. Purslane
4. Anise	21. Horehound	37. Quince
5. Bayberry	22. Hyssop	38. Red clover
6. Cardamom seed	23. Jujube	39. Red raspberry
7. Cayenne pepper	24. Licorice	40. Rose
(African)	25. Lily of the valley	41. Saffron
8. Chamomile	26. Linseed	42. Sandalwood
9. Chickory	27. Lobelia	43. Senna
10. Comfrey	28. Manna	44. Squaw vine
11. Coriander	29. Marshmallow	45. Sumach
12. Cowslip	30. Masterwort	46. Valerian
13. Cassia	(imperial root)	47. Violet
14. Dill	31. Melilot	48. Water lily
15. Fennel	32. Mugwort	49. Wild rue
16. Feverfew	33. Myrtle	50. Wormwood
17. Frankincense	34. Peppermint	

These can be purchased in one-ounce quantities, along with glass bottles with childproof caps (highly recommended!) for approximately $30 at today's prices. These basic fifty will allow you to compound most of the formulas listed in this book, as well as most other well-known remedies that may be passed along to you.

There are other herbs that some may feel should be included in this basic list, and with experience you will undoubtedly arrive at your own favorites. A useful book containing information on suppliers of herbs, especially hard-to-find botanicals, is Richard Heffern's *The Herb Buyer's Guide* (New York: Pyramid Books, 1973).

Directions for Herbal Preparations

Once you have determined a formula you wish to use and have obtained the herbs, it is important that the formula be prepared properly. For the purpose of convenience, I have used some terms which apply to the fixing of herbs, such as *infusion, pomade, tincture,* and so forth. Rather than give a complete set of instructions of preparation in each case, this "shorthand" of herbalogy allows us to give a one- or two-word directive that applies to any herb used. In addition, different directions are sometimes given, due to the ability of one process to extract one active principle from the herb, while a different action will result in removing another element. For example, an infusion of lobelia will give a mildly sedative effect, whereas a tincture of lobelia can produce an emetic effect.

Below are some of the most commonly used concentrations:

Capsules These are made simply by taking the herb in powdered form, or ground finely, and placing in a gelatin capsule. These are available in sizes from 00 to 4, with 0 and 00 being the sizes most often used for herbs. Capsules make herbs with an acrid taste or unpleasant oils more palatable.

After making the capsules, be sure to keep in a safe container, accurately labeled, including the date of preparation.

Conserve (Sweetmeat) A soft mass of the herb mixed with sugar or honey. We usually recommend turbinado sugar, although date sugar works as well. Sugar burns at a higher temperature in the stomach than does honey, but the medicinal property of honey is consumed faster than sugar.

To make a conserve, such as rose conserve, gather fresh rose petals and add sugar in the amount of three times the weight of the petals. Mash it together with a mortar and pestle until congealed. If honey is used, roll the mixture in a little orris root powder to keep it from sticking to your hands.

Decoction Many roots and barks, as well as some stems and flowers, must be boiled for some time before their active principle is extracted. The proportion usually is one teaspoon of the dried herb to one cup of water. Always use stainless steel, glass, or porcelain vessels to make decoctions. A coffee percolator may be used to make a decoction. If none is available, boil the substance for two minutes, then simmer for twenty minutes covered. Let cool, add honey or other flavoring if desired, and use.

Essence   Obtain one ounce of the essential oil of the herb **and** add four drops to one pint of pure water. This is sometimes very expensive for true natural essential oils (pure amber, for example, costs approximately $400 per ounce) and so often synthetic oils are sold as "natural." Of course, synthetics do not have the same healing properties and can be used for aromatic purposes only. If the true essential oil can be obtained, dissolve one ounce in one pint of cider vinegar (if it is to be preserved).

Fomentation   Dip a cloth in an infusion or decoction and place over the area to be treated.

Infusion   Take one-half to one ounce of the herb (leaves, flowers, root, or bark) and pour one cup boiling water over the herb. Let it stand for three to five minutes. Infusions should be consumed or applied while fresh, and the portion not used should be discarded. The infusion is usually the weakest form in which an herb will be used.

Jujube   A paste made of equal parts of gum Arabic and sugar.

Mother's milk   Mother's milk has natural antibodies and is the most complete food, capable of sustaining the life of an infant for several years. You can of course obtain fresh mother's milk directly from a nursing mother, if available in your family. If not, the local chapter of La Leche League can usually supply frozen mother's milk. Also, most health food stores carry a product made in West Germany called Euglan Töpfer Forte, which is a cultured (bifidium) preparation on a base of mother's milk. It is in powdered form, and can be mixed up and used in place of fresh mother's milk.

Oil   This must be made from the part of the plant that contains the particular oil desired. The best oils of peppermint, for example, come from the leaves. The most aromatic oils are usually derived from the blossoms of flowers. The basic ratio is three or more ounces of an herb to one pint of olive oil, which is the recommended base because it does not easily become rancid and can be kept a long time. Never use mineral oil, as it is not safe for internal consumption. Heat the herb in the oil at about 140°F. Afterwards, strain and bottle. Another method is to simmer up to a pound of the herb in a pint of water until the oil is extracted—usually four or more hours.

Ointment   *See* Salve.

Oxymel   This is a standard preparation in the Eastern pharmacies. It is made simply by mixing five parts honey to one part vinegar.

Pomade   *See* Salve.

Plaster   Bruise the leaves, root, or other part of the herb and place between two pieces of cloth. Moisten slightly and apply to the surface you desire to cover.

Poultice   The purpose of a poultice is to apply heat, draw out toxins, and soothe an inflamed area. Some work by producing a counterirritation, some draw blood to the area, and some relax and soothe. Simmer two ounces of the herb in half a pint of water for two minutes, then pour the entire solution (without draining) into cheesecloth. Apply the herb poultice directly to area, covering with cheesecloth and a second layer of clean cloth.

Salve   (also called *ointment* or *pomade*). The base for a salve is usually one of the following: almond oil, coconut oil, wax, or Vaseline. You can also mix some of these together to make a more readily absorbed salve or to slow down absorption. Vaseline is not soluble in water and is recommended when it is undesirable to allow rapid absorption, such as for application to any of the mucus membranes.

   Begin with two pints almond oil or other melted lubricant. Add about a pound of the herbs in their natural state, a pound and a half of vegetable lard, and two ounces of beeswax. Place in a stainless-steel, earthenware, or glass container and put into the oven for three to four hours at about 150°F. Check the herbs from time to time to see that they are still submerged and not turning brown or brittle.

A stronger ointment can be obtained by using more of the herb, which is also required if dried herbs are used (increase to a pound and a half of the herb). You will be able to tell when the active principle has been extracted by the dark color of the oil base. Cool, strain, and put in wide-mouth jars or bottles for use.

A quick method of making a salve is to take one part each of almond oil, honey, and beeswax and add one part of the remedy you wish to use. Heat the lubricant, and mix in the herb (powdered finely). Let cool until it gels and apply. Another method of making salve is to boil the ingredient herb in water for twenty minutes. Strain off sediment, add fresh herbs, and repeat the boiling process (cover while boiling). Strain again. Add the resultant decoction to half a pint of olive oil and simmer until all the water has evaporated. Strain again. Add enough beeswax or resin to solidify. Melt over a low flame and keep stirring until thoroughly mixed.

Suppository This is a preparation of herbs mixed with a suppository base such as cacao butter or glycerinated gelatin and molded into special shapes for insertion into the rectum, vagina, or urethra. The suppository bases are solid at room temperature but melt at the temperature of the body. Suppositories should be stored in a refrigerator, especially during the summer.

Suppositories are made in the following sizes and shapes:

rectal—tapered, about 2 grams
urethral—pencil-shaped, pointed on one end; 7 cm in length, 2
    grams
vaginal—oval, 5 grams

You can purchase the base from a pharmaceutical supply house or pharmacy or make your own by lightly heating one of the bases mentioned above and adding the recommended amount of finely powdered herb. Dosage varies according to age, sex, condition, and similar factors.

Syrup.   A syrup is a thick liquid preparation made by dissolving sugar into water, decoctions, infusions, or the like. To make a syrup, first make a decoction (or other liquid base) and settle off any sediment. Then, to every pint of herbal liquid, add one and three-quarters pounds of turbinado or date sugar. Place in a stainless-steel pan and heat until the sugar is melted (there will be some scumming, which can be taken off as it cools). Cool and store for later use.

Tincture   Take one ounce of herb, powdered, add four ounces of water and twelve ounces of cider vinegar. Let stand two weeks. After two weeks, add one teaspoon of glycerin, stir thoroughly, strain off liquid, and seal in bottles. If the herb is weak in medicinal power, the original amount of the herb may be increased from one ounce to two or four.

Water   A water solution in which herbs are soaked is a weak infusion. These can be made by taking half a pound of the herb, blossom, or green part, or other vegetable, placing in pure water in direct sunlight for four hours, preferably from midmorning until after the sun has passed its zenith in the sky. Properties for healing are extracted from many grains and seeds in this way. If you can't make a pure water for any reason, an infusion is an acceptable substitute. This is the manner in which the Bach flower remedies are made.[1]

Notes on Preparation   While it may seem time-consuming to make a tincture, for example, it should be done if that is what is called for in the remedy. If you don't have time to make a tincture (two weeks), most herbs are available in ready-made tinctures from health food stores, botanical firms, or homeopathic pharmacies. Remember that it is important to use the

---

[1] Dr. Edward Bach, a London physician, devised thirty-eight flower remedies corresponding to the "thirty-eight main negative states of mind," which he divided into seven groups: fear, uncertainty, insufficient interest in present circumstances, loneliness, oversensitivity to influences, despondency, and overcare for the welfare of others. He often used two or more of the remedies in combination. The Bach flower remedies are sold in 4-ml bottles, which is an ample supply as the dosage is only a few drops of each mixed with a glass of pure water. The distributor of these remedies is the Dr. Edward Bach Healing Centre, Mount Vernon, Sotwell, Wallingford, Berkshire, England.

herb as recommended, for there is often a difference in the properties, depending on how it is prepared. For example, a weak infusion of hops will extract aromatic properties, while a stronger infusion will extract the bitter tonic principle. A decoction will extract the astringent properties. People using herbs for the first time are often disappointed when they "don't work." Each preparation will give a specific result: an herb will not yield the same properties from an infusion as from a decoction.

Dosage   Most single and compound herbal preparations given in the Formulary are accompanied by proper instructions for dosage. It is very difficult to give an exact dosage to be followed in every case, as each person has a different body, so these that follow must be taken as an average. The rule adhered to by the great herbalists of all times is to begin with the smallest dose first and work toward gradually larger doses, *if needed.* The dose is also to be altered depending on the age of the person. A child of ten usually will require half the adult dose; a child of five can generally be given one-quarter of the adult dose. According to Dr. John Christopher, it is wise to give nervous, high-strung persons smaller and more frequent doses. Also, in applying diuretics, it is better to begin with small doses, so that the kidneys are not forced when in a weakened condition. The instructions for preparing the various forms of medication are given in the Formulary. Follow them carefully.

General Dosage

Capsule   This is completely dependent upon the age, sex, general health, and nature of the condition. A general rule is to give capsules as follows:

Number 0:   Three, three times per day, with meals.
Number 00:   Two, three times per day.
Number 4:   One or two, five or six times per day.
Number 2:   Two at wake-up, two at bedtime.

Conserve (Sweetmeat)   Use amount specified in Formulary, or one tablespoon with tea after meals.

Enema   Ratio for most herbs is one and one-half tablespoons to each pint of water (do not give more than one pint at a time for children or one quart for adults).

Essence   Dose variable. Consult Formulary.

Fomentation   The cloth should be wet enough with the fomentation so that the fluid does not run off the body; keep damp and change every half hour to hour.

Infusion   One cup, three times per day is the general rule, although there is great variation in application of infusions.

Oil   Oils are quite potent, and should not be overdosed. One drop to one tablespoon is the quantity limit for internal consumption. Externally, you may wish to dilute a pure flower essence with a less expensive oil such as olive oil for massages and similar application.

Oxymel   One mouthful as a gargle.

Plaster   Make up to one-half-inch thick and large enough to cover the affected area; plasters build up heat, so must be used with care and in consideration of the general state of the person.

Poultice   If the herb is not too expensive or potent, use profusely.

Salve   Use enough to cover the area, but not so much that residue is left on the skin.

Syrup   According to size and age, 1 teaspoon to 1 tablespoon.

Tincture   The Formulary recommends various doses. One ounce of tincture is equal in strength to approximately one ounce of the powdered herb, so three drops will be equal to a half cup of tea. Unless used to provoke vomiting (lobelia), or unless otherwise directed, always mix one teaspoon of tincture with at least one cup of water.

Methods of Improving and Adjusting without Reaching to the Stomach

We must remember at all times that the stomach is the seat of disease. When digestion fails, disease follows sooner or later. It is for this reason that we often desire to use a method of correcting a part of the body without sending substances into the stomach, which may further disturb a digestion already upset. A review of the wide range of methods of correcting balance without ingesting anything follows:

1. What is smelled, wet, or dry.
2. What is soft and sweet-smelling, and put in a bottle for inhaling the vapor.
3. What is dropped into the nose.
4. What is sniffed into the nose.
5. What is dropped into the throat.
6. Ground substances put on the teeth.
7. What is dropped into the ears and other orifices.
8. What is rubbed on the body, oils, washes, and salves.
9. Warming the body by steaming.
10. Alternating warm and cool compresses on the body.
11. Rubbing wet substances on the body.
12. Injecting liquid into the intestine, anus, bladder or womb.
13. What is shaped and inserted into the anus or vulva.
14. What is ground in water and used to bathe the eyes.
15. Soaking a tampon with herbal preparation and inserting in anus or vulva.
16. What is ground and poured on wounds.
17. Substances burned and the vapor inhaled.
18. Pouring herbal preparations in water and sitting in it.
19. Boiling herbs and placing the feet in the bath.

Inasmuch as many ailments arise from an imbalance of the *senses*, it is often sensible to try and apply a remedy to the affected sense area; that is, the mouth, eyes, ears, or nose. The many available avenues of treatment *before* any medicine is consumed are important to keep in mind, as we so often think that we must *eat* something, medicinal or otherwise, in order to become well. Remember, fasting is the best medicine!

Fevers

It has been explained in the chapters on the origin and progression of illness that fever is a normal function of the body by which heat is developed to fully process and eliminate excess matters from the body, so that congestion and impairment of organ function does not occur.

In natural medicine, fevers are studied from this point of view, and different fevers are classified according to their characteristics.

Day fever This type of fever lasts only one day. Mental or psychic causes include illusions, mental anguish, anger, happiness, pain, wrong food consumption, flu, catarrh, excess fluid in the body, and so forth. If the fever is more related to the essence, or purely mental causes, the heart can also be felt to become hot. The temperature of a day fever, while elevated, is not "burning," as the heat is when caused by injury. There are no signs of infection present, and the fever usually goes away in twenty-four hours unless it changes into another form of fever.

The remedy is to consider the cause and remove it as much as possible, especially emotional stress. Reduced intake of food will allow any obstruction of the narrow veins to be cleared away, and the fever will pass. Warm baths are especially useful to soothe and relax.

Mixed fever of the blood One blood fever is due to simple increase of internal heat, which gradually increases until fever comes. There is no infection.

Another blood fever is caused by infection, which can be known from putrid odor of urine and feces and other signs of infected blood. The blood must be purified, which can be accomplished by using the remedy suggested in the section on the blood humour. If the blood is thick, soften it with oxymel. If impurities still remain along with the fever, give this remedy: 20 drams green chickory water boiled for ten minutes. Scrape off the foam that appears on the top of the mixture and add 15 drams of oxymel to that. If there is coughing with the fever, add water of quince seeds and syrup of violet. When there is thin blood, it can be thickened by drinking plenty of jujube tea or syrup. Plum juice is very good for this purpose too.

Fever of yellow bile If bile enters the veins and becomes infected, fever comes and goes every other day and signs of phlegm are present. If the corrupted bile gets into the veins surrounding the heart and stomach, the signs are severe. This is the kind of fever present in typhus. If the bile is outside the veins, the signs of phlegm fever appear every other day.

The bilious substance needs to be made cold and moist. If there is constipation, the substance is still in the veins.

Usually the body can correct the corruption by itself, and thus the signs of bile fever do not last more than one week. If there is phlegm mixed with it, the course of the fever is two weeks.

The general treatment is to alter the diet to cold foods and to use bile and phlegm purgatives.

If the person gets chills and trembles, he can be given oxymel and warm water to throw off the bile by vomiting. If there is grumbling in the stomach, give laxatives. If the urine is retained, give diuretics. If there is much phlegm, do not overdo the use of cold foods and herbs. Generally, if you do not know for certain the origin and characteristics of the fever, do not try to cure it with herbs, for the body can do this well enough on its own. Merely try to keep the avenues of elimination open.

Phlegm fever The phlegm can also become infected, and this infection is carried inside the veins around the heart and stomach, which results in the fever.

If the substance is infected outside the veins, the person does not tremble or have chills, but feels weak once or twice a day.

However, if it is salty phlegm (which can be tasted), there are chills and gooseflesh. The sign of sour phlegm is that the chills and coldness are very severe; sweet phlegm is accompanied by less cold signs and has the shortest duration.

Most phlegm fevers are accompanied by constipation, which can be removed by giving a half dram of rose preserve (jam) in the morning, followed by 10 drams of oxymel.

The general regimen to remove phlegm fever is to take oxymel for a week, along with honey water in which infusion of hyssop and a little anise and peas have been cooked. After a week, the phlegm should be ripened, and an emetic can be given to remove the phlegm. Oxymel with warm water will accomplish this purpose; it should be given on the day the fever returns. Chickory-root enemas help keep the bowels clear of mucus.

Black bile fever   The sign of this fever is that it becomes severe every two days, and the nature of the corruption is determined by which day the fever returns—that is, on the fourth, fifth, seventh, ninth, or tenth day. The most frequent black bile fever returns every four days. It is caused by unnatural or corrupted black bile (every phlegm that becomes hot turns into black bile). The fourth-day fever is often the result of chronic conditions and passes quickly, usually within a few hours. It will return five or six times in a period of two weeks, disappear for a month or longer, then return.

The treatment consists of obtaining a complete evaluation and detoxification of the body. Iridology may help to discover in which organs the corrupted substance has settled.

On the first day the fever returns, go on a fast: no food or water is best, but especially avoid cold water. No fresh fruits or gas-producing foods should be eaten. Detoxification for several months may be necessary to cleanse toxic buildup.

NOTE: It does happen that while one kind of fever is active in the body, another one arises at the same time; this is called interference. Another variation is that while one fever leaves, another kind comes, which is called partnership. These complex fevers need careful treatment by a healing practitioner.

Hectic fever In this form of fever, the heat reaches the heart and the natural moisture of the body begins to be destroyed. When it becomes chronic, hair loss may result. The first sign is a mild fever, and then after eating a meal, the fever goes high. The pulse is weak but constant. Give herbs and foods that moisten and cool (see Chapter 4). The diet must be regulated most carefully to provide only the best nutrients for the body. Buttermilk is helpful in hectic fever. As far as possible, reinforce all the important organs of the body, especially the brain, liver, heart, and intestines.

Typhoid and cholera fever The body develops fever to repel bacterial infestation as well as to purify its own by-products. The signs of typhoid fever are great restlessness, backache, itching nose, tears, and disorientation on waking up from sleep.

Cholera fever can be fatal; as with typhoid, it should be treated by a qualified physician. Since these diseases are so rare in the United States that treatment is omitted here. Inoculations against both these diseases are available and should be taken if you are traveling where outbreaks of cholera and typhoid are known to exist.

The Healing Crisis

Every imbalance that is corrected by the body's own healing mechanism has five steps: addiction, growth, end, decline and crisis.

The stage of addiction is the period when the body is exposed to the actions or substances that are ultimately the cause of the disease. The time of growth is the period during which the substances are accumulated—or for germs, when they grow without the body's own defense mechanisms being brought into action. The time of crisis is when the body acts to repel the cause of the disease, whatever its nature. The crisis may happen at the end stage of the disease and be quite sudden, or it may appear mildly from time to time even during the growth period.

The crisis occurs at these varying periods, due to the nature of the substances and the means being used to correct them. The body is never idle, but sometimes must assume a status of stand-by, just waiting for the substance to be refined enough to be thrown off.

The disease can be considered an enemy, and the physical health is compared to a king guarding his territory. The day of crisis is compared to the day of battle. On fighting day, the king has a complete control over how he will use his fighting forces to repel the enemy: suddenly attacking, mounting all the troops for a big attack, or splitting them into fighting factions.

As on a real fighting day, both sides provide the weapons of the battle, and the terrible sounds of cries of battle can be heard. The person feels fear and anxiety, hears voices, and rough and abrupt movements shake his body.

On the day of the healing crisis, the person should never be stimulated, for if the stimulant works in the same way—in agreement—with the natural healing mechanism, it will weaken the natural disease-repelling force. If the stimulation works against the natural repulsive faculties, the body's nerves and inner systems will become confused and Nature is prevented from her complete action: the substance is not taken out fully and the disease is not completely eradicated. Thus, on the day of crisis, avoid herbs that provoke diarrhea or vomiting or other stimulation, and avoid as much as possible feeding the person.

Crisis, in terms of substance repulsed, has five modes: vomiting, diarrhea, nosebleeding, urine, and perspiration. Crisis by urine and perspiration is incomplete because the thin substance is thrown out and the thick one remains. The crisis by vomiting, nosebleeding, and diarrhea is complete.

If the crisis is to happen during the day, the signs appear the night before, or vice versa. Each crisis is preceded by its own signs. For example, the sign of crisis by vomiting is asthma, change in breath rhythm, bitter taste in mouth, cardiac pain, stomach convulsions, lowered pulse, trembling of the lower lip. The signs of diarrhea are intestinal pain, heaviness of body, stomach gas, backache, colored feces, and grumbling intestines.

The signs of crisis by nosebleeding are dull sense of hearing, ringing in ears, tears, nose-itching, and beating of veins in head. Signs of urine crisis are heaviness of urinary bladder, thickness and excess of urine, bright color of urine on fourth day of illness, and full crisis on the seventh day.

You should pay attention to the process of crisis, to see if the substances are expelled with force. If not, the elimination is incomplete and a doctor must be consulted to complete the repulsion of the substances.

The correction of disease occurs from the top of the body downward and from the inside outward. Thus, the first sign of a crisis often is headache, lastly diarrhea. Furthermore, in the process of the correction of the body, the order of signs is acute, subacute, chronic, and degenerative. The first signs in the acute stage are heat, swelling, redness, and pain. If the body can repel the substance or correct the inharmony of this stage, it will. If not, the disease will be driven further into the body and become chronic. This stage may last weeks or years, depending on many factors. When the chronic stage is not corrected, organ damage occurs and the signs of degenerative disease are present.

It is easy to see that the time to correct any condition is at the first time of seeing any sign of imbalance. It will take less time and less effort and will be healed more quickly. In correcting during the chronic and degenerative stages, the disease must retrace back through each of the stages it went through in arriving at an advanced condition. This is why, when people are able to recover health via natural medicine, the last signs of healing are often the *same ones* that occurred when the disease first began. Those trained in natural therapeutics know how to recognize these signs and effectively manage the healing crisis.

The Four Qualities of the Body Reviewed

In a previous chapter, the four qualities of heat, cold, moisture, and dryness were given in conjunction with the four elements. Now we must understand them as biological functions in order to arrive at the means to correct them when they go out of balance. We shall discuss them in terms of excesses.

Excess of heat   Heat is warmth, and its signs are thirst, burning, yellowness or redness of a part of the body. If the cause of an excess of heat is an excess of blood, the symptoms are dizziness, yawning, frequent naps, dullness, sweet taste in the mouth, skin redness, inflamed tongue, boils, excretion of blood from the gums and nose, and tiredness and pain all over the body. If the cause of excess of heat is oversecretion of bile, the symptoms are yellowness of the skin, tongue, and eyes; a bitter taste on the tongue (which may also be coarse and dry) and nose; extreme thirst; loss of appetite; and prickling sensation.

Excess of cold   In the simplest sense, cold means lack of life or the life force. The symptoms are unnatural lack of thirst and pale color. If the cause of coldness is an excess of phlegm (due to faulty elimination), the symptoms are paleness of the body; soft, loose, and cold skin; poor digestion; sour belching; oversleeping; excess salivation; runny nose; and insensitivity to hot liquids in the mouth and nose. If the cause is an excess irritation of the tissue membranes (itching, scaly patches on skin, etc.), the symptoms are loss of weight, thickness of the blood, irritation, prickling sensation in the upper part of the stomach, and false appetite.

Excess of moisture   The symptoms of excess of moisture in the bodily system are weakness of the extremities and anything that suggests lack of dryness, such as moist skin, excessive salivation, clammy feet, and the like. If an excess of moisture is combined with an excess of heat (or an excess of coldness), the symptoms will be the same as for the primary condition of excess, already given.

Excess of dryness   The symptoms of excess of dryness are loss of weight, dryness of the skin and other parts, and dullness of the eyes. It should be recalled that none of these qualities exists by itself, but rather in a constantly changing and self-balancing system. The term for the interconnection of these four qualities is *humours*.

The four humours In terms of anatomy, humours, or plexus, may be defined as the entire network of blood and lymphatic vessels and nerves. One site of such an interwoven arrangement is the *solar plexus*, with which we are all familiar. There are four types of humour in the inner systems of the body, and an excess of any one or more, or lack of the same, can cause disease.

The overall strength of the body is derived from the balance of these four kinds of humour: blood, phlegm, yellow bile, and black bile.

When in a harmonious state, the four systems are of the following constitution:

Blood humour is moist and warm.
Phlegm humour is cold and moist.
Yellow bile humour is dry and cold.
Black bile humour is warm and dry.

The charts on pages 104–105 summarize which of these four systems is dominant by the signs that occur in the individual.

Adjustors

Herbal preparations that bring about a change in the humour to the normal state are called *adjustors*. These include consumed foods. Each adjustor will be explained separately since each one affects one of the humours.

Adjusting the Blood Humour

There are four abnormal conditions of the blood: (1) increase in quantity; (2) thickness; (3) thinness; and (4) infection. The blood should be adjusted whenever there is a change from the normal state.

To correct thick blood Thick blood can be caused by black bile being mixed with it, which in turn causes canker. The herbs that correct thick blood are black cherry juice, anise juice, and

HUMOUR DOMINANT

EVIDENCE	Blood	Phlegm	Yellow Bile	Black Bile
Aspect: General physique	Good	Effeminate; bones slender, joints well-covered	Lean, joints large	Emaciated
Color	Flushed	Pale and weak	Yellow tinge in skin and eyes	Dusky; whole body seems dark and hairy
Feel of the skin State of the skin	Firm Reddens on rubbing; boils	Soft and cool		Flesh hard Skin rough, liable to dark eruptions and ulcers
Hair		Absent on chest	Hairy	Hairy
Surface veins	Full	Constricted	Thick and hard	
Vegetative faculties Mouth	Tendency to canker sores	Abundant sticky saliva	Bitter taste	
Tongue	Red		Rough and dry	
Nostrils			Rough and dry	
Pulse		Soft, tends to be slow and infrequent	Rapid	
Urine		White		Dark-colored or black; dense

Sensitive faculties				
Special senses: taste	Unusual sweetness in mouth, senses dull		Bitter taste	Sense of burning at mouth of stomach.
Appetite for food			Poor	Depraved; faulty cravings
Appetite for fluid		Absent unless salt is taken, esp. in old people	Thirsty	
Muscular tone	Weariness not accounted for by exercise	Flaccidity of limbs		
Dreams	Sees red things; blood coming out of the body; swimming in blood, and the like	Sees waters, rivers, snow, rain, cold, thunder	Sees fires, yellow flags; objects not yellow appear yellow; a conflagration; hot bath; hot sun, etc.	Fear of darkness, of torture; terrifying black things
Movements (gestures)	Yawning, stretching			
Rational faculties: Signs	Reaction time slow; always drowsy	Sleepiness, laziness, tiredness, lassitude	Dull	Sense of anxiety; wakefulness
Abnormal phenomena	Nausea; Sense of weight in back of eyes and temples; Blood flows out readily from nose, anus, gums	Weak digestion and acid eruptions	Nausea; Yellow and green bile and acidity; Gooseflesh; Severe diarrhea	Splenic disorders often occur, also ulcers

honey, which remove the canker and soften the blood. A second cause of thickened blood is phlegm, which causes the blood to lighten in color. Since the blood is being mixed with phlegm, a phlegmagogue is first given to ripen the phlegm, and after that a diuretic is given.

To correct moist blood   Often moist blood is also a sign of phlegm mixed with the blood. It is necessary to take the phlegm out of the system, which can be done by a three-day detoxification followed by a laxative. To dry the moisture, after detoxification, the person should take sweet basil in foods and tea, and it is also advisable to massage the body.

To correct soft blood   This is often caused by excess yellow bile being mixed with the blood, which can be detected by the presence of a yellowish foam riding on the surface of the blood. This biliousness can be eliminated by giving a laxative and giving a preparation composed of jujube syrup, one part; yellow dates, one part; and infusions of lentils and chickory seeds, two parts.

To correct infected blood   Infected blood is caused by the introduction of germs. Any excess of phlegm, when infected by germs, causes fever. (Phlegm is never infected unless it causes fever.) To lower a fever caused by infection, give seeds of chickory, seeds of lettuce, coriander, rose tea, lemon juice, honey with sandalwood syrup, and similar cold foods. Anything that becomes infected becomes hot from the exertions of the body to throw off the germs.

Adjusting the Yellow Bile

There are several ways in which yellow bile can be affected, resulting in a change in humour: *softened moisture* can mix with yellow bile; *thick moisture* can mix with yellow bile; *black bile* can mix with yellow bile. There are two kinds of hot yellow bile: (1) normal bile mixes with hot bile to produce thickened bile; and (2) normal bile mixes with burning bile to produce white bile. The only difference in these two conditions is the degree of heat, which is less in the thickened bile. Any bilious condition marked by production of heat should be corrected by giving cold foods and herbs two or three times per day.

Single herbs that correct yellow bile humour   There are many herbal remedies for simple biliousness, and the correct one must be given according to judgment about the individual person and overall condition.

Cottonseeds:	Boil cottonseeds and take the water, or drink the water with the seeds. *Never pound or apply a mortar to cottonseeds, as they become poisonous.* Also American cottonseeds are full of deadly poisons from chemical pesticides. Make sure you get uncontaminated seeds.
Quince seeds:	Boil about thirty quince seeds and give the resulting liquid. Do not use seeds of sour quince, especially if there is a cough.
Chickory seeds:	Boil half an ounce of chickory seeds and consume the liquid. If seeds are not available, take the raw plant and boil it. (Never wash chickory for it will remove the active ingredient, and make it ineffective.) Boil the water two or three times, until there is a soft feeling to it. Then give the water alone, or add a little honey and vinegar. This is very effective in refining the blood.
Coriander:	Take half an ounce of dry coriander, soak in water for an hour, and add a small amount of turbinado sugar.
Sandalwood:	Grind sandalwood (one-sixth of an ounce), mix with water, and consume. It will lower severe temperatures. White sandalwood is better than red for this purpose.
Watermelon:	This and other melons, cucumbers, and various kinds of vinegars are effective adjusters of biliousness.

Compound medicines that adjust yellow bile   Syrup of sandalwood, plums, and violet flowers are mixed in equal parts and the aroma sniffed into the nose. Rub a portion of the mixture over the body. This adjusts yellow bile and lowers the temperature as well.

Adjusting the Phlegm Humour

Imbalance of phlegm occurs in five forms: (1) a little blood is mixed with phlegm, called *sweet phlegm;* (2) burning bile is mixed with phlegm, called *salty phlegm;* (3) a slightly raised temperature affects phlegm, called *sour phlegm;* (4) a little black bile is mixed with phlegm, called *coarse* phlegm; (5) the phlegm is composed of more water than mucus, called *tasteless phlegm,* which is the coldest kind of phlegm. The signs of these can usually be determined by taste as phlegm is ejected via the nasal passages or throat. A test for phlegm imbalance is to take the person's index finger and bend it forward quickly at the midjoint. If the color takes four or five seconds to return, the phlegm is unbalanced.

Single herbs that adjust phlegm   These are anise, cinnamon, valerian root, large black raisins, cardamom, and mugwort. If the phlegm has a foul odor, no hot medicine should be given. Sometimes it is advisable to combine the remedy for biliousness with one of the above herbs.

Compound medicines that adjust phlegm   Equal parts of ginger and garlic can be used when there is no foul odor to the phlegm and there is no fever. If there is fever, take equal parts of agrimony and rose petals pounded with turbinado sugar; add honey to make a paste. Take a teaspoonful with tea three times per day.

Change in course of phlegm   A buildup of phlegm occurs because there is an unnaturally high degree of black bile, burning blood (high fever), burning phlegm, or burning yellow bile. Any phlegm that burns causes canker. Burning means that the phlegm is soft and that the "thin" or watery parts of the phlegm are consumed, and the remainder is thickened in a way that changes the nature of the phlegm. It does not mean, however, that it is literally burned up or destroyed.

External phlegm adjustors Often due to complications of digestion or loss of appetite during illness, it is necessary to adjust the phlegm by giving an external application. The list given earlier indicates the many methods that can be employed.

Inhalations for hot imbalance In every case of excess heat, there are aromas useful to correct the inharmony. White sandalwood ground in vinegar, coriander, and rose petals is quite good. If the person is sleepless, do not use vinegar. Smelling cucumber cut into small pieces, other fruits, and cold flowers—all are useful. If the odor of coriander is offensive, smell a decoction of pumpkin seeds instead.

Inhalations for cold imbalance Smells that are useful for cold inharmony are musk, ambergris, cinnamon, castoreum, clove, and saffron. They can be used as much as needed.

Ripening of Phlegm

Phlegm takes nine days to become ripened. The formula to ripen phlegm is: plum, 20 grains; jujube, 10 grains; cowslip, 2 grams; mint, 2 grams; anise, 2 grams. Cook these together in a pint of water for ten minutes. Give a half-teacup portion with tea, three times each day.

The meaning of ripening is becoming softened and easy to expel. It doesn't mean that the substance becomes cooked, as noted earlier. It is impossible for phlegm to be expelled before it is ripened, for it is within the nature of the body to ripen phlegm and all other humours. Naturally, if the body is overcongested to begin with, this process is slowed down or impaired and medicine becomes necessary to assist this process.

Every phlegm should be ripened according to its nature. Thus, thick phlegm should be made thin, and that which is hot cooled, and so forth. Mild heat makes the phlegm soft, and cold makes it thick. If a fever appears the first day of illness, it is because of a condition of the blood, not phlegm. Thick blood is known from all signs of coldness or wetness, thin blood by signs of hotness and dryness. If the thickness of the blood is due to phlegm, care must be taken to ripen it according to the prevalence of phlegm (i.e., hot, cold, moist, or dry).

Ripening Biliousness

The compound to ripen biliousness is jujube, 7 grains; violet, 2 grams; rose, 2 grams; chickory seeds, half-ground, 3 grams; chickory root, half-ground, 2 grams. Soak this compound in water for twenty-four hours. Rub and filter off liquid. Give one teaspoon of the liquid three times per day, after meals. This preparation can also be boiled and taken as a tea.

Biliousness will become ripened in three days if it is pure; if impure, it will take five or more days to become ripened. Pure black bile is ripened in fifteen days.

Purgatives and Laxatives

Once phlegm or bile is ripened, it must be removed. A purgative is that which removes substances or accumulations in the further reaches of the extremities and veins. A laxative is that which removes what is in the stomach and intestines. When giving a purgative, it is important to ripen first, as instructed above. The effect of a purgative is opposite to that of a laxative. Therefore, the ripening medicines include laxatives as it is better to give both at the same time. Purgatives containing laxatives may be given to pregnant women, children, and the elderly, but should be administered only after consultation with a physician who is familiar with the entire health picture of the person. Laxatives are good for swellings of the intestines.

The general purgative remedy recommended is a decoction

of cassia and the soft part of a cucumber soaked in rose water, or just plain warm water. If there is a fever, add chickory seeds to it. If the intestine is swollen, add gentian. To make the preparation stronger, add purgative manna to it. If the person has weak intestines, never give purging cassia without almond oil, because the intestines are already soft. The dose for the purging cassia medicine is 4 grams. Doses in excess of this can be harmful.

General Directions for Purgatives

When the purgative is seen to be effective, do not give any cold water following. When the purgative is given, have the person try to sleep. When the bowels must be moved, purify the bathroom afterward by washing with marshmallow infusion, or wash down with plain warm water. If the purgative does not work, do not repeat the dose the same day. It is better to follow with a suppository. If a strong purgative has been given and the person becomes senseless, induce vomiting and call a physician. If the temperature goes very high in the stomach and intestines, give a decoction of seeds of quince.

Sometimes a medicine to adjust the temperament is recommended following a purgative. Soak half an ounce of sweet basil in one pint rose water for one hour. It is a refreshing drink.

A purgative that is not complete is harmful, for the toxins which have been stirred up are loosened in the body. If a patient is strong, a purgative can be given daily; if weak, every other day. If dysentery results and makes the person weak (and there is no high temperature and fever), give yogurt and rice. If there is fever, give seeds of sweet basil browned in safflower oil along with plantain seeds browned in the same way.

Biliousness Purgatives

The single herbs are violet, plum, fumitory, rose leaves, tamarind, and purgative manna: one-quarter ounce in a cup of water to make a decoction. Some of these have an immediate effect, some do not. Make a decoction of one and take once.

The compound preparation for biliousness purging is composed of

plum, 15 grams
fumatory, senna, 3 grams each
jujube, 9 grains
seeds of chickory, 2 grams
cassia, from 10 to 15 grams

It may be boiled in a tea or mixed with two ounces of honey and eaten. If it is boiled, add 1 gram of almond or violet oil to it.

Phlegm Purgatives

Lobelia, comfrey, and wild rue in single infusions will take out phlegm. Although there are three kinds of phlegm, there are no herbs that will act upon each of them singly. The compound preparation for removing phlegm is to make an infusion combining lobelia, comfrey, and wild rue. If there is a fever with chronic coughing, this formula is useful:

plum and jujube, 20 grams each
hyssop, violet, and fennel, half-ground, 3 grams each
large raisins, 15 grams
dried fig, 7 grams
licorice root, partially crushed, 4 grams

Boil them in three cups of water. Boil down to one cup, filter and add cucumber, rose hips, and sugar (5 grams each) to it, boil for ten minutes, and filter again. Then add a gram of sweet almond oil and drink.

A pounded preparation also useful for removing phlegm is made as follows: ginger powder, sifted, 3 grams; sea salt, half a gram. Drink with cold water. The salt can be replaced with sugar, but mastic herb must then be added, and it should be drunk with warm water instead of cold.

Black Bile Purgatives

The formula recommended for correcting black bile is: senna, 7 grams; rose hips, 4 grams; cowslip, mint, 3 grams each; anise, 2 grains; ginger, half a gram. Boil for five minutes, filter, and consume. It can be made stronger by adding half an ounce of juice of aloe vera.

Enemas

Enemas and suppositories often have good effects on dysentery. The use of an enema is not very popular, but, as noted in the chapter on detoxification, it is recommended and very useful.

Suppositories

If a laxative is tried and doesn't work, use a suppository. Also, if the person is afflicted with colic, it is not proper to give an enema or laxative before trying a suppository. In the case of constipation, laxatives and purgatives take time, and a suppository often works much more efficiently. Unless you have an urgent need, do not use suppositories frequently, as they may cause hemorrhoids. The suppository that removes colic and cleans the stomach is: violet, 2 grams; marshmallow, 3 grams; senna, 5 grams; salt, 1 gram; juice of cucumber and sugar, each 10 grams. Shape them into suppositories as long as the index finger. (If it is to reach the colon, it must be longer.)

The suppository to be used after purgatives is composed of soft soap from olive oil, marshmallow, and sea salt, each 2 grams; beet sugar, 5 grams. A piece of pure Castile soap cut into a piece the size of a date stone has an immediate effect as well.

A suppository used for children and debilitated people is composed of beeswax, 2 grams; salt, one-half gram. Pound and shape into suppository form, lubricate with rose oil, and use.

Herbs to Provoke Emesis (Vomiting)

The procedure of emesis is a great cleansing of the entire body. It cleanses the stomach and alimentary canal and clears out much accumulated superfluous matters. An emetic, properly taken, leaves one feeling very clean and light, and tingling to the tips of the extremities. If a need for emesis is felt, take soft foods for one day before procuring emesis. If the temperature is a little low, lubricate the body with sweet oil. On the day of emesis, eat only soft foods, such as rice and broth. If one has trouble vomiting, it is better to take warm baths for three days prior, rub oil on the body, and drink oily soups.

At the time of drinking emetic, rub the waist and abdomen. Some say that to vomit while standing and lowering the head takes the phlegm out of the deep part of the stomach, and vomiting is easier in this position. Rather than taking an overly strong emetic, it is better to repeat the procedure. In the summertime, wash the eyes and face with cold water after vomiting. In winter, wash with warm water. In both seasons, gargle with honey and vinegar after vomiting. After gargling, take four grams of aloe wood or mastic herb mixed with a small amount of sugar and rose water. If the stomach is upset after vomiting, chicken or miso soup is good. If pain is felt in the sides or chest, rub rose oil over the torso.

Emetic for Biliousness

Add 40 grams of vinegar to 140 grams of an infusion of spinach water or barley water and consume to provoke vomiting.

Emetic for Phlegm

To remove phlegm, give a preparation of radish seeds, 2 grams; common dill seed, 1 gram; salt, half a gram. Pound all these together and mix with honey. If vomiting does not occur within a few minutes, follow with small amounts of warm water.

Emetic to Remove Biliousness and Phlegm

The compound is composed of vinegar, 40 grams; salt, 8 grams; radish juice, 140 grams. Another formula is made of water lily root, partially crushed, and common dill seeds, 20 grams each; seeds of barley, 12 grams. Boil them in three cups of water until reduced by half. Filter and add enough cider vinegar to make it sour.

Diuretics

A diuretic is that which throws out substances through the urethra and also purges the veins of the urethra. Diuretics are not recommended in conditions in which there is prevalence of phlegm, unless an enema is given first. Furthermore, diuretics are not advised unless the ailment is moist, according to the humoral concepts (dropsy, rheumatism, and the like).

Cold Diuretic

Oxymel or any of the following single herbs in decoction will produce elimination: chickory seeds, cucumber seeds, purslane seeds, and watermelon seeds.

Hot Diuretic

For hot imbalance, a decoction of these herbs will produce diuresis: celery seeds, anise, mugwort, hyssop, and carrot seeds.

Mild Diuretic

A general-use diuretic is made in this way: partially crush 2 grams of anise and boil in one cup of water. Filter the liquid and add 3 grams each of powdered melon and cucumber seeds to it. Sweeten with sugar and drink. It is useful to simply relieve urine.

This concludes the theoretical aspects of natural medicine.

What follows is a complete formulary of specific remedies for many conditions. The foregoing herbal formulas have been given, relating to the body humours, inner systems, hot and cold imbalances, and the like, as these will often be recommended in the formulas that follow, to be used before or in conjunction with a specific regimen of herbal preparations.

It should be borne in mind that a qualified physician or other healing professional should be consulted if one chooses to use any of these formulas for any ailment. As each person is totally unique, it is possible that some herbal remedies will work differently in different persons.

How to Apply Cupping

In some of the conditions described in the Formulary, the recommendation for treatment includes cupping. These ailments include stomach problems, abdominal gas, bruises, abscesses, and others.

Precautions

Sites and conditions to avoid are skin conditions, all bony prominences, and sites prone to cramps, areas showing any superficial blood vessels and much hair growth; also tumors, lymphatic nodes, and the abdomen, chest, and breasts of pregnant women.

The *hakims* say that cupping should not be applied to children under two years of age or to persons over sixty. The best time of cupping is the sixteenth and seventeenth days of the month, three hours after sunrise. Also, be careful not to apply cupping for extended periods on the nape of the neck, as it induces amnesia.

Technique

Have the person lie down on a bed or massage table, in case he faints during treatment. If the person feels unwell doing the procedure, discontinue immediately. Select cupping sites or swollen spot.

The duration of application should be from ten to fifteen minutes, or at least enough time for reddish stripes to appear in the cupping area.

Equipment

Use a glass cup, such as a shot glass, (1 to 1½ inches in diameter) on healthy young people or persons in generally good physical shape. Use smaller ones for the elderly, weak, or chronically ill as well as for children.

Application

Hold a flaming alcohol sponge (ball of cotton saturated with isopropyl alcohol) with a pair of forceps or large tweezers and quickly apply the flame to the inside of the cup, then remove. At this time, due to the flame, the air inside the cup has become less dense, and the cup placed instantly over the selected spot will attach itself firmly to the skin, because of the atmosphere pressure outside. This method is quite safe.

Removal

After ten to fifteen minutes, press the skin around the edges of the cup to remove it. When air from the outside enters the cup, it will fall off by itself. Do not use strong pressure on the cup to prevent cutting the skin.[1]

[1]Information on cupping from *A Barefoot Doctor's Manual: The American Translation of the Official Chinese Paramedical Manual*, tr. by John E. Fogarty (Philadelphia: Running Press, 1977), pp. 80–81.

The Well-being of Children

Raising Children

Children are extremely delicate and elegant in body, temperature, and temperament. Their temper, as it adjusts to growth, should be kept very balanced and moderate, as the temper is such that it responds quite rapidly and easily to events going on about it. The reason for this tendency to moods and activities about the child is the prevalence of phlegm in large quantities in its body, and the shifting weaknesses and softness of the body parts as they undergo growth.

Therefore it is necessary to keep children away from all extreme effects upon their sensibilities—such as severe anger, great fear, staying awake for extended periods, or also sleeping for a long time. These things spoil childrens' happiness and can lead not only to unhappiness of the child but also to the beginnings of disease.

It is merely common sense that parents, doctors, or anyone caring for a child should be aware of what a child likes and dislikes. Things that are obviously harmful to a child should be kept away, regardless of how strenuously the child desires them; but if there is no harm in what a child desires, it should be given readily to the child, for it contributes to a happy disposition and good nature. A sense of humor should always be behind the guidance, whether bending to a child's desires or keeping harmful objects or activities away from it. Usefulness and harmfulness are of two kinds: one is useful to the body; the other is useful to essence and soul. But what is useful to the body is health itself, for if the body is always wracked with illness and upsets, the temper will be bad, because of the relation between body and the essence.

Bad temperament of the kind that is considered hot from a humoral point of view is manifested in a child who is reticent to speak, standoffish, wanting to spend long periods alone, and often feeling afraid. Bad morals or defective character can often be traced directly to an upset of temper in early childhood. "He's got a hot temper" is often used to describe an unpleasant adult—forceful and selfish, immature and impulsive. But the badness of temper is the result of a bad emotional environment in childhood, one that exposes a delicate child to extremes of anger, sadness, and noise. The nature of a human being is to be independent, happy, and balanced. In addition to proper nourishment of food for a balanced body, the spirit and soul must also be nourished by keeping the essence healthy. Severe anger is one of the basic causes of bad temperament and other indispositions, because it so easily throws off the balance between body and essence.

When a child rises from sleeping, it is an ideal time for a bath, which should be with lukewarm water. After the bath, the child should be left free to play with other children of his own age, in games that are not harmful (for about an hour or a little longer) to consume the natural energy that has built up during rest. A child should not often play with others who are older or younger, because with younger children he cannot use his abilities to their full extent and because with older children he is not really qualified in skills, and thus becomes frustrated and disposed to feeling failure. During adolescence, the child should be fed after an hour of play a light meal or snack—as much as it needs to increase growth. If it wants to play again after that, the child should not be restrained; but if the child wants to sleep, that is fine as well. After sleep, a lukewarm bath will refresh the child at a time when his mood is calm. For a daily schedule, the conditions of play and food should be considered in relation to time of day, the season, climate, altitude, and similar factors.

At the age of four, a child should be taught the matters of manners and politeness, and the formal aspects of learning can begin. From the age of seven onward, teaching of politeness should increase. It is important that the teacher be a model as well. While the influence of parents is needed and ever-present, someone outside the basic family structure can be considered for the child's instruction in morals, attitudes toward life, religious ideals and ethics, manners of dealing with parents, teachers, pious persons, relatives, friends, peers, and those who are younger than the child. The child should be taught in a conscious way how to visit, meet, and speak with each of these societal categories and how to gather people together in meetings. According to the child's age and understanding of matters related to his religion and sciences, things that will help him progress in more formal studies must be taught. The child should only be given instruction in an amount that can be held in its mind and remembered without strain, so that the child does not become tired, bored, or angry. Whoever is selected to teach the child should speak to the child with kindness and mildness. If the child becomes tired or displeased, the teacher should let him go, to walk around or play for a time.

At the age of ten, the frequency of bathing a child can decrease, and the meaning of disappointments, politeness, general education, and self-discipline should increase. Toward the age of fourteen or fifteen, which is nearing adulthood, the child should be introduced to mild fasting and other self-disciplines, as the phlegm which has been in its system is being used up and the extreme agility of play and the powerful exertions are being exhausted. It is at this time that parts of the body are hardening and stiffening into the bone structure and musculature of adulthood; this can be experienced as growing pains. If, during this period, a child neglects its studies, it should be punished. Children's temper is much hotter during this stage if not brought under control by mild, enforced hardships. This is the last stage on the road to adulthood, and if the child does not encounter such hardships as mild and fair punishments, in later life, when tempers and powers are weakened, the child will be prone to increases in the balance of moisture. Even at this stage, moisture can become a problem, and should be cured as the situation requires.

The foregoing brief presentation of the stages of growth of a child shows how to keep a balanced body and spirit, which will contribute to a happy, well-adjusted childhood into pre-adulthood. In some cases, either through inharmonious outside influence, poor diet, or other factors, disease occurs. The following three sections are devoted to the most common of these disturbances, with remedies given to restore balance to the child's physical and spiritual system.

Infancy

1.1 Skin

From the time of birth, the child will be exposed to many hot and cold substances injurious to an infant's sensitive skin. Therefore, an effort is made to condition the skin against this. Bathing in a salt water solution (one teaspoon to a quart of pure water) each day for the first several weeks will help to accomplish this purpose.

1.2 Sleeping quarters

Babies must be placed in rooms that are airy without being too cold. Since their eyes are very sensitive to extremes, keep the drapes closed or windows covered to prevent extremes of direct light. Even a gloomy atmosphere is all right for the first month or so. During sleep, the head should be raised slightly higher than the rest of the body, and the baby should be checked from time to time to make certain that its limbs are not twisted into unusual positions.

1.3 Bathing

Hold it by the right hand, so that the left arm is across its chest and not hanging down over its stomach. After washing, bounce the palms of its hands and soles of the feet up and down gently. Dry gently with a soft cloth, first placing it on the stomach, then on the back, gently singing to it all the while. Put a drop of sweet rose oil or other pleasant oil into the nose, and dab a little on its eyelids.

1.4 Nursing

If at all possible, the baby should be fed from its own mother by nursing at the breast. A mother's milk is most like the nourishment the infant received while in the womb—the menstrual nutrients—and it is these that are changed into the milk after delivery. It is best suited to the baby. Infants will naturally suck at the breast if the nipple is pinched and placed between its lips. Allow the baby to nurse two or three times per day at first, but it should not be allowed to take too much. Remember that the mother has just undergone a great upheaval in her own system, and it is good to allow her a few days to recover some balance.

1.5 Strengthening the Constitution

Gentle rocking movements, humming, lightly singing, and cooing at the baby are customary and soothing for the baby. The movement benefits the body; the melodies benefit the mind.

1.6 Inability to Nurse

Nursing problems are discussed in the Formulary. The La Leche League in your city will be glad to provide free assistance during your nursing if any problems occur. Frozen milk is usually available to keep up nursing even if the mother is ill. Powdered mother's milk is available in most health food stores.

1.7 Test for Good Milk

Test for the proper consistency by allowing a small amount to run over the fingernail; it should be thin and flow easily. If you tip your finger upward slightly and the milk does not flow back down, it is thick. Place an ounce or two of your milk into a glass, drop a pinch of myrrh into it, and stir together. The milk will separate into the liquid and "cheesy" part, which should be about equal in quantity. Breast milk should be white (not grayish or yellowish), of good odor, and taste a little sweet (not bitter or salty), with little or no foam in it.

1.8 Diet

If the milk is thick, the mother should drink a little honey with vinegar (two ounces of vinegar and a tablespoon of honey). Wild marjoram, hyssop, thyme, savory, and oregano should be added to foods. If the milk is thin, the nursing mother should avoid exercise for a while and eat foods that thicken, such as meat broths and bread soups. Adequate rest is vital.

1.9 How Long to Nurse

Most natural mothers will desire to nurse a child for two years, if possible. If other foods are to be added to child's diet, they should be added gradually over a period of months. This will allow any allergic reactions to be noted and enable identification of the foods that cause such reactions. Weaning must not be abrupt, but allow the child to withdraw over several months. After the first teeth appear, more substantial foods should be considered. If indigestion or flatulence occur, all foods should be stopped for at least eight hours, and a warm, soothing bath should be given to the baby. If the infant at weaning time keeps crying and asking for the breast, make a poultice of one ounce of myrrh, and add an ounce of very smoothly ground pennyroyal, and apply as a paste to the breast and let the baby suck at that.

1.10 Walking

There is no rush to compel a child to sit up or walk. By forcing a child prematurely into postures for these acts, great strain is placed upon the bones and muscles of the back. Be especially careful that the child is not allowed to climb up on a high chair or other place and fall off. Childproof the home when the child begins to move about.

1.11 Teething

At the time when the child's teeth are coming in, keep all hard things out of its mouth, for by gnawing on them the substance that is becoming the teeth may be worn away and dissolve, leaving deformed teeth. Allow the child to chew on a piece of arrowroot instead, and rub the back and neck with warm oils after the teeth do break through the gums. A few drops of the same oil may be dropped into the ears. As soon as the child realizes it has teeth, it may try and bite its own fingers, so give a stick of dry licorice root to chew on. Rubbing the gums with salt and honey will take away some of the pain of teething. When most of the first teeth are in, they should be rubbed several times a week, at the base of the gums. New teeth sometimes seem to itch. Let the child chew on a dill pickle.

1.12 Inflammation of the Gums

This condition, called gingivitis, may occur while the teeth are coming in. Swelling may also occur around the juncture of the jawbone. You should press firmly against the swollen parts in the mouth, or along the outside of the jawbone, and rub the gums with ten drops of oil of camomile added to honey.

1.13 Diarrhea

Many babies develop diarrhea during teething. Some healers say it is due to the ingestion of salty saline matter excreted by the gums during dentition. Whatever the cause, it interrupts normal function, and, if severe, must be treated. Suggested treatments include applying a plaster of caraway, rose hips, anise, and celery or parsley seeds (about equal parts) to the stomach. A plaster treated with infusion of rose leaves and caraway works also. If the skin loses its elasticity and the baby becomes senseless, it is an emergency. Take the baby to a doctor or hospital.

1.14 Constipation

A suppository may be used, made from honey cooked over a low flame until it becomes thick enough to shape into a "finger" for insertion into the anus. Adding a little honey or rice-bran syrup to the milk also improves bowel movement.

1.15 Incessant Crying; Loss of Sleep

The causes of incessant crying are heat, cold, bugs (flies, fleas, etc.), hunger, thirst, retention of urine, and retained feces. For retained feces, the nursing mother should eat some prunes or add a tablespoon of olive oil to her diet twice a day. If sleep must be had, make a decoction of lobelia, add a half teaspoon to eight ounces of water, and allow the infant to drink an ounce or two. Or add one drop of oil of peppermint to eight ounces of water and let it drink as much as it wants.

1.16 Earache

This is caused by excess moisture in the brain, or trapped gas. It may be treated by making an oil from turbinado sugar, lentils, myrrh or cedar seeds; put one or two drops into the ear.

1.17 Difficult Breathing

Rub olive oil on the base of the ears and on the tongue. You can also press the back of the tongue down to cause vomiting, which will ensure that there is no obstruction of the airway. Water may be dropped into the mouth, drop by drop, as well as a little linseed and honey to suck on. NOTE: Loss of voice in infants is due to constipation. Give cabbage juice by mouth or rectum.

1.18 Cough

Some healers advise that the baby's head should be bathed in plenty of warm water. A steam vaporizer will also work well. Put plenty of honey on the tongue, and cause the baby to vomit and expel excess mucus in the stomach. A few grains of the following may be added to the milk: gum arabic, quince seed (set twenty or so seeds in water for half an hour and a gummy substance will form). Give a half teaspoon of this mixture to the baby, or brown sugar.

1.19 Severe Vomiting

Feed three grains of clove, very finely ground.

1.20 Hiccough

Feed a piece of fresh coconut dipped in sugar.

1.21 Colic

The baby writhes and cries. Apply hot water bottles to the stomach, and give peppermint water.

1.22 Skin Rash

In all kinds of skin rash of unknown origin, treat by bathing in soothing waters; you may use any of these: rose, myrtle, tamarisk, marjoram, peppermint, or almonds. Also recommended is a decoction of dates and figs, mixed in water of fennel seeds. When the rash has developed fully, bathe in rose water, then rub rose oil on the affected parts.

1.23 Fevers

As explained elsewhere, fevers are not necessarily a negative sign, but they can sometimes quickly get out of hand with small babies, or even children for that matter. Liquid calcium will quickly lower a fever, about a teaspoon added to mother's milk or water. Cool baths can be used to bathe the child to keep a fever from getting too high. Apply cold cloths on its head, chest, and extremities between baths. See the following sections and index for specific diseases accompanied by fevers.

Nervous Disorders

Some people call these conditions epilepsy, while others think it is a kind of epilepsy followed by burning fever. Still others feel that it is not truly epilepsy, but some disorder related to epilepsy.

The signs of this affliction are that the child falls down abruptly, senseless, and the feet become twisted, the eyes squinted, and foam appears at the mouth. When the child is restored to his senses, it weeps a great deal, will not take the breast or bottle, and is quite restless. The cause of this illness is an accumulation of wind, or air, in the head, such that the scalp becomes slightly enlarged and the spaces between the front teeth can be seen to widen. This may be due to the evaporation of milk in the child's stomach, from which excess air is carried via the bloodstream into the brain and affects the cells, causing a kind of simulated spastic hyperventilation. Sometimes a parent will miss the signs of the disease and call it a temper tantrum.

If there is no deterioration of the brain cells, the child recovers quickly. But, if untreated, this affliction can indeed lead to full and more frequent seizures, sometimes ending in death. The sign of the illness increasing is that the attacks come more frequently, one after the other, each time more violent than before. Regardless of the severity, the cause is the excess of air being carried to and filling the brain cavity. If the attacks come with less frequency and intensity, it is a sign that there is a decrease of the air and its assimilation.

The first prudent measure is to avoid eating foods that cause evaporation and spoil very easily—such as eggs—overeating, intake of air with breast or bottle, and emotional disturbance such as anger and fear. Standing in places where strong winds blow, and other extremes, should be avoided. Constipation also worsens the condition, as it blocks the natural flow-off and excretion of waste from digestion. If the condition worsens, the palms and soles of the feet should be massaged, and any influence that causes anxiety should be screened from the child. In extreme cases, the hands and arms should be bound to the sides to prevent self-injury. The foregoing should alleviate mild cases.

If the illness lingers on or becomes complicated (plethora of phlegm is a sign of increase of illness), further measures should be taken such as increasing the child's water intake, rubbing the body with mild salves, and softening the abdomen by using suppositories or feeding laxatives. Good laxatives for this consist of decoctions extracted from boiled chicory, fish eggs, rose, jujube, senna, borage, or plum—with a few grains purging cassia or purgative manna dissolved into the mixture. This should be filtered and mixed with sweet almond oil, warmed and eaten, one teaspoonful, with liquid.

As the condition itself is brought on by what really is staleness of the mind, or entry into the brain of rotted matter, however minute, the best thing to refresh the mind is to obtain some milk from a nursing mother. Gently tilt the head of the ill child back and drop some of this fresh milk into the child's nose. Also, a piece of clean cloth can be soaked in the mother's milk and put on the top of the child's head like a scarf. Other efficacious means are to rub its body with flower oil and butter. These applications are useful in reducing tension. When phlegm is present in large amounts, it is important to keep the child warm. A most effective medicine for phlegm is to take 2 grains each of wild thyme, pennyroyal, and cumin. These should be ground and dissolved in mother's milk, shaped into pills and eaten, one with each meal.

Use of suppositories is considered useful in remedying constipation. Boiled gum of plum with sugar in lukewarm water also helps soften the bowels and produce movement. The vapor of juice of aloes and saffron will cause sneezing, thereby loosening the muscles; the vapor of mustard soaked in vinegar will have the same effect. Any milk from a nursing mother used in the foregoing medicines should be pure and her diet should also be free from foods producing gas and phlegm.

Coughing

The reflexive action of the lungs and throat known as coughing is often taken for granted as a natural effort of the system to expel foreign matter. However, whatever the underlying causes, coughing can be the precursive sign of more serious diseases in formation, and in every case disturbs the normal harmony of breathing. Breath is the bridge to life, and its frequent disturbance in childhood can upset the entire mental and physiological process of development.

There are several conditions that produce coughing. The first cause is penetration of smoke (from fire, stoves, or cigarettes) into the throat. Remove the child from the source of the smoke, and to alleviate the cough give the child a small amount of honey.

A second cause of coughing is dust. Shield the child from the dust, and oil the breast and throat with almond oil or violet oil. If the child is old enough to eat solid foods, it should be fed oily food and gargle with milk.

A third condition of which coughing is a symptom is dryness and coarseness of the lungs. The remedy is again rubbing the throat and the breast with oil and wax and feeding a decoction of seeds of quince with a little sugar. If the child is bilious, give black mulberry water or black cherry decoction. If the child is old enough to eat regular meals, the medicine should be given prior to meals. Sometimes an enema or a laxative is helpful.

A fourth cause is flu. Children are especially susceptible to flu, and it is generally known in its milder, natural form as a children's disease. The medication for coughing without running nose (or before it can be called flu) is to make a decoction of jujube, plum, violet, borage,or dry hyssop, and give for three days.

Coughing pills made from dried egg white ground with a little sugar and dissolved in mother's milk can be given at night. Give the child one or two small balls. In the morning, feed the child a sweet paste of almonds and walnuts, and keep the chest warm by rubbing with lanolin to stop the coughing.

If there is constipation, give pulp of purging cassia or purgative manna with almond oil added to it. If the pulp of purging cassia does not work to relieve the bowels, or if the child refuses the cassia because of its taste, add a few leaves of senna to the decoction; rub the chest with a salve made of almond oil and wax.

To prevent phlegm from developing when the weather is cold, keep the child from breathing cold air, talking too much, and drinking cold water. Rub castoreum on the temples, palms, soles of feet, and in the nose. If there is a lot of phlegm, mix a tablespoon of honey in one cup lukewarm water and feed it to the child. If that doesn't remove the congestion, take a dab ot honey on the tip of the finger, add a dash of confectioner's sugar, and rub it on the end of the child's tongue to draw the congestion out of the chest.

It helps to expel the phlegm if it is ripe, which will happen automatically if the cause of the coughing is the phlegm. To assist expulsion of phlegm, mash a grain of gum Arabic or a dozen seeds of quince with one gram of sugar, mix with mother's milk, and feed to the child. Syrup of hyssop seed has a great effect as well. The best diet for this condition is vetch or one of the rice dishes in Chapter 4.

If the coughing is followed by phlegm, the child shouldn't be given foods that are dry and produce many calories, especially when the child is feverish. All efforts should be made to control the fever by lowering the temperature, which alone may cause the phlegm to disappear.

If the coughing and phlegm persist, set up a steam vaporizer and place the child near it in the morning. Because the nostrils are blocked by the cold air of dawn, the inside of the chest is warmed by this vapor, and thus the congested matter that is causing the flu is dissolved and the flu will disappear. Keep the head covered as much as possible.

If the coughing is followed by both phlegm and fever, give the following: quince seeds, violet flower, jujube, and borage. If you want to soften the stomach and help to promote digestion, dissolve 3 drams of cassia in this mixture and feed to the child. If the child is under seven years, give three teaspoons; if older, a little more can be given. Vinegar should not be consumed, nor should calorie-rich foods. To stop coughing, especially at night, grind equal parts of bitter almond, gum Arabic, and clove.

CAUTION: Opium, while illegal in the West for general consumption, has found its way into some homes. It is very effective in stopping coughs, as well as relieving pain and promoting sleep and rest. However, when the person has coughing followed by phlegm and fever, opium will increase the temperature and dry and harden the phlegm, which may result in emphysema, typhoid fever, swelling of the lungs, or death. In January 1978, a young couple in Arizona gave a very small quantity of opium to their child to stem a cough and promote sleep. The child never awoke. As it is an illegal substance and the dangers inherent in its ignorant use great, it is not recommended. Great care must be taken when giving any psychoactive or central-nervous-system agent to a child. In all cases, a doctor or experienced medical practitioner first should be sought to correctly diagnose the disease.

Measles and Smallpox

Measles is a disease characterized by small red boils the size of millet. Before the red spots can be seen, the skin swells in small bumps; the skin then wrinkles, and finally small boils develop on the surface of the skin. These boils contain a type of blood that is not mature or has not been properly assimilated into the blood composition. Usually, the boil dries to an outer scale which separates and falls off. Smallpox is a disease characterized by boils as big as lentils, sometimes bigger, filled with rheum. The appearance of measles or smallpox is preceded by fever, accompanied by pain in the back region, itching, scratchy nose, redness and tearing of the eyes, nightmares, burning sensation of the skin, and/or prickly feeling over the whole body. Some children are also affected by coughing, earache, emphysema, and hoarseness.

Fever in measles is milder or less hot than smallpox fever, and pain in the back, if present, is less severe than with smallpox. Also, measles appear suddenly, "breaking out" more or less at once, while smallpox appears over a three- to seven-day period. Measles are usually more dangerous to the life of a child, especially the worst type of measles.

A severe infection of smallpox is indicated by pox that are connected one to another and appear as one piece, or great numbers of pox on chest and abdomen, or pox that ripen late or ooze blood. If the smallpox appear followed by fever or if the fever does not weaken immediately after the smallpox appear, both are signs of severity, especially the latter sign.

The signs of the mildest forms of measles and smallpox are that the child is fully conscious, no change or coarseness in voice, and the appetite for food and water remains stable. The cause of smallpox and measles is the boiling of the blood, due to the rawness and presence of phlegm that is in the nature of children. Congestion of the blood and other bodily systems results in this boiling of the blood (as evidenced by fever), and the skin boils are the signs of the completion of the boiling process. Rarely, pox or boils appear without the attendant fevering and boiling of the blood.

Prevention of Measles and Smallpox

Measles (to some extent) have been controlled or eliminated by effective inoculation programs of public health authorities. However, some people do not have access to even rural health care (in the United States as well as many underdeveloped nations), so the following measures are recommended for diet and prevention of these afflictions, especially during the summer when these diseases are prevalent.

In general, these foods, all of which increase biliousness and heat of the blood, should be avoided: milk, sweet peas, syrups, meat, and eggplant; honey, figs, dates, melons, and grapes should not be eaten by mother or baby. Instead, foods that keep children in a good mood should be given, such as juice of pomegranate, tamarind juice, and other *fresh* juices. Children should be kept from running and walking in direct sun for long periods, sitting close to fire, and any other activities that overexert or overheat their systems.

The best foods during summer months are cold and sour vegetables such as spinach, pumpkin, and purslane, and occasionally beef with vegetables and vinegar.

The best precaution against smallpox and measles, especially when outbreaks of these diseases occur, is to stop children from eating candies and dry foods and other foods that cause high-caloric burning inside the body.

When either of these diseases appears, it is necessary also to purify the blood. This can be done by giving special diet and drinks. If the child is full of phlegm, it must be cleared out, and bad or difficult digestion should be avoided. Since smallpox has been eradicated in this country by vaccines, only information on measles will be given.

The following recipes are given as the most frequently mentioned preventive medicines for measles and smallpox:

Red rose, 3 grams
magnesia, 3 grams
white sandal, 2 grams
chicory seeds, purslane seeds, pumpkin seed stones, and lettuce
seeds, 2 grams each
gum tragacanth, 1 gram
camphor, .5 grams.

Grind all together, then sieve and form pills with infusion of fleawort. Adults take two grams, children half a gram. During the warmer summer months, showers of cold water sometimes prevent appearance of smallpox and measles or greatly lessen the severity if contracted.

Fevers of Measles

The fever of measles is usually very hot. The child's mouth is bitter, the eyes yellow, and the urine rose or red-colored. The remedy is to first reduce phlegm by mild laxatives; if the fever is mild, a pain reliever can be given, such as noncoal tar-base children's aspirin. Some physicians forbid using medicines that make the blood cold or thick when there are measles *with no boils on the skin.* They reason that the boiling of the blood at this time is a process of nature to remove waste matter from the system. Medicines that thicken the blood, and thus slow the elimination process, are acting against the natural bodily function.

When boils do finally appear on the skin, cover the child's body with soft clothes and keep warm. The temperature of the room should be moderate. The boils will surface quickly. Burn sandal incense and make a slight vapor of camphor to strengthen the heart and mind, and stimulate the natural process of transfer of matter to the surface of the skin. The sign that the matter is thickened is that more boils appear on the chest and do not completely disappear after four days. The sign that the boils are blocked below the surface of the skin is that the skin is rough and very little sweat comes out.

The general condition of the child must be taken into account in treatment. For example, if the pulse and breathing are normal and there is no fainting or loss of consciousness, and if the temperature is normal and there is no blackness of the tongue, make the room a little warm. Do not give cold water, but rather lukewarm water, perhaps with a little anise water from time to time. This formula is useful: mother's milk, 4 grams; lentils, 4 grams; gum Arabic, 3 grams. Mix them all together and boil until half of it remains. Give it, a teaspoon at a time, every few hours. The medicine is more efficacious if you add 2 grams of rose water, a few ground figs, and 2 grams anise to the mixture. An alternative: boil a few figs and add a pinch of saffron to it. You can put a hot-water bottle under the child's blanket to vaporize and open the pores. The child's head should not be under the blanket, for if the vapor goes into his nose, it will cause itching and restlessness.

When the boils have appeared completely, the child should be given cold juices, as much as is readily accepted. Special attention should be paid to the condition of the stomach and bowels. When the boils have completely come out, protection of the eyes, nose, throat, lungs, and intestines is necessary. If boils are appearing in these areas, they will be slight and light in color.

1 Protection of the Eyes

Put a drop of the following mixture in each eye: sumac soaked in rose water, filtered and added to one grain of camphor, three times daily. Another good mixture is water of fresh coriander seeds, with seeds of sour pomegranate, and rose water in equal parts; put these drops in the child's eyes. Both medicines have the same effect. If the eyes are swollen, put a bandage over them after using the medicine to cure the swelling. If the child becomes very nervous or restless, untie and remove the bandage from time to time.

2 Care of the Nose

Drops of vinegar with rose water or flower oil with a little camphor should be rubbed up inside the nose. Apply cold compresses over the nose area. If the blood coming out of the nose is blackish and the child will not sleep and has severe coughing, the illness is severe and medical aid should be sought at once.

3 Care of the Throat

When the boils appear on the surface of the skin, or even during the preceding time of fever, it is good to give pomegranate (this should not be given to children under two years old). The child should chew the seeds and swallow the juice. Three useful gargles:

A decoction of sumac, red clover blossoms, and lentils boiled in rose water.
Iced water mixed with rose water.
Black cherry juice.

4 Care of the Lungs

When the boils appear, if there is no hoarseness in the throat, take the temperature and check whether the bowels are moving fast or slowly. If the temperature is high and the bowels are sluggish, give water of quince and fleawort with sugar in small doses, and put ground almond in the child's mouth. Licking this medicine can be tried if the child won't take it into the mouth. If, in spite of the temperature, the bowels remain loose, take gum Arabic, almond, pumpkin seeds, and seeds of cucumber (one-quarter ounce each), fry each one separately; then grind them together and fry in an infusion of fleawort. Let the child lick this medicine. If the temperature is not high and bowels not soft, give fresh butter with sugar, gradually and in small doses.

5 Care of the Joints

For sore joints and boils grind sandal, clay, and red clover blossoms with a little camphor, add a little rose water and vinegar, and rub onto joints. If a boil appears and opens by itself, no further treatment is necessary. If it doesn't open, a doctor may have to pierce the boil to let out the rheum.

6 Care of the Intestines and Bowels

Sometimes, although the boils of measles seem to be drying and clearing, their remnants are left under the skin and transferred to the intestines, spreading the infection there. To avoid this complication, give the child a syrup of myrtle, pills of magnesia, and quince juice, *at the time the boils seem to be drying.* Care of the intestines is very important at this time.

When the boils have completely appeared, cold juices should be given, and constipation and looseness of bowels regulated. Do not give any laxatives at this time. If the stomach is loosening on its own, do not give anything that will block up the bowels too quickly.

7 Diet

Generally, children affected with measles should be given cold and dry foods, such as barley composite, which can be prepared as follows:

> Take one pound of barley, split the corns into halves, grind, and remove skins after one hour. Then fry the remaining split barley, put through a sieve, and add lentils and juice of sour pomegranate, green grapes, or rhubarb.

If the child's bowels are not soft or loose and there is a feeling of coarseness in the chest and throat but no temperature elevation, give the above mixture with sugar syrup, but do not make it too sweet. *Never feed sour foods* if the bowels are constipated.

If the bowels are loose and the temperature high, and the chest and throat coarse, fry the above composition; cool and refry *several times,* and mix with magnesia. If there is severe diarrhea, give water of fried barley and ten grains of pomegranate in equal parts.

Severe symptoms of measles indicate that the internal temperature is too high, which leads to burning of the blood and biliousness. Everything given should be cold and juicy, like the water of boiled barley. Vinegar can be added to the barley if there is no coughing. If there is coughing, give purslane, melon water, pumpkin water, and similar foods, but these should not be given with vinegar.

Recommended Readings

Eiger, Marvin, and Sally Olds. *The Complete Book of Breastfeeding.* New York: Bantam, 1972.

Elolesser, Leo, Edith Galt, and Isabel Hemingway. *Pregnancy, Childbirth and the Newborn: A Manual for Rural Midwives.* Mexico: Inter-American Indian Institute, 1973.

Khan, Hazrat Inayat. *The Sufi Message,* Vol. III. London: Barrie & Jenkins, 1971.

Myles, Margaret. *Textbook for Midwives.* New York: Longmans, 1974.

Sousa, Marion. *Childbirth at Home.* New York: Bantam, 1976.

Section 2

The Head

General Considerations

Every physician knows that if the subject of disease is looked into deeply enough, every ailment can be said to originate in the mind. Dr. Lewis Thomas, President of the Memorial Sloan-Kettering Cancer Center in New York City, has suggested that despite the astounding advancements in removing most of the plagues of humanity, such as tuberculosis, smallpox, polio-myelitis, and other scourges of humanity, people are today more fearful about their health than ever before. He claims that the majority of people who go to a doctor's office have nothing organically wrong with them. The problem is rather that 75 percent of the people visit the doctor because they are fundamentally unhappy. What does this say about us and the times we live in?

Despite the tremendous research applied to all areas of human knowledge, the human mind cannot be fathomed, even in a small way. There are no methods known to control with repeated accuracy the focusing of the mind on negative aspects of one's life. No doubt, the sixty million legitimate prescriptions for Valium and the tens of millions of other drugs given to raise the threshhold of anxiety are mute testimony to the complete failure of modern science—and medicine—to deal with the underlying true causes of human illness.

To the great healers of the past and present who truly understand human health, there is only one way to assure a stable mind, and that is by gaining contact with and discovering the full magnificence of one's immortal Being. It is immaterial

138

what name or term is applied to this phenomenon. It is real and often accounts for spontaneous cures of the most baffling diseases.

There are probably as many paths to such awareness as there are people, and it is vital that people must acknowledge this reality as something more important than any other aspect of their daily lives. Meditation, yoga, breathing exercises, shiatsu and other massage techniques, Rolfing, body balancing, and hundreds of alternative modalities of health building are really efforts to silence and harmonize the "outer" person, so that the mind can be brought into balance. Violence, fear, worry, avarice, and sirens throughout the night can easily be called to task as causative agents for much of the disease produced by irregularity of living habits. All of the recognized prophetic religions of the world contain programs of organized study and application of the divine principles of fit conduct of human life on earth, and, as such, are worthy of the most intelligent and careful study. Mahatma Gandhi once wrote of his study of all the religions of man that their essence could be summed up in these words: "Live and let live." This is the vital prescription and message of our time for the relief of suffering humanity.

2.1 Headache

Headaches are often caused by eyestrain, stress, or the obnoxious noises of city life. Rest in a darkened room and drinking a cup of camomile, valerian root, or peppermint tea often relieve a simple headache.

Headaches are also caused by unbalanced humours. Check for signs of a dominant humour. If the cause of headache is inharmony of the blood humour, cupping on the back of the head is useful. After cupping, give sour lemon. If the cause is biliousness, take an enema and add to the formula sandalwood and coriander, about 5 grams each. If the cause is phlegm, use the phlegm adjustor, followed by boiled anise seeds mixed with honey, which should be rubbed on the neck and shoulders. If the cause is black bile, adjust by giving a black bile purgative and massage the neck and shoulders with sweet almond oil.

Washing of the feet and zone therapy (see Appendix II) is

the best method for every kind of headache. Do not rub the head. Although this will produce immediate relief, its long-term effect is negative. It is always better to use foot reflexology.

2.2 Headache Caused by Heat or Cold Intemperament without Prevalence of Phlegm

If caused by heat, give foods from the list of cold foods in Chapter 4. If caused by cold, do the opposite. If the headache is linked with fever, cure the fever first. If the headache occurs on one side of the head and not the other, this formula is useful: gum Arabic, 1 gram; cannabis sativa, ½ gram; saffron, ¼ gram. Mix these with the white of an egg or rose water. Spread this on a piece of plain paper and stick to the temple on the affected side. It is especially useful if placed on a throbbing blood vessel.

2.3 Use of Cannabis Sativa and Narcotics for Headache

It is not at all recommended to use marijuana for recreational purposes or as a regular part of one's regimen. Ill effects are

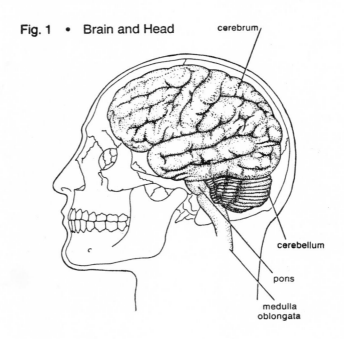

Fig. 1 • Brain and Head

quite well known in cultures that have a history of centuries of consumption by the populace. In a few cases, since it is available and legal in some areas, it is recommended in the minute doses noted, as the method of choice as opposed to using a more potent drug.

If this or other narcotic drugs are to be used in any case at all, side effects can be minimized by taking a small amount of saffron along with it (note formula in 2.2). Some also recommend bathing the head with rose water; it should be applied copiously to wet the entire head.

The most intelligent book on drugs and altered states of consciousness is *The Natural Mind* by Andrew Weil (Boston, Houghton-Mifflin, 1974), although the book is really about much more than drugs. Using his background as a Harvard M.D., Weil traveled widely throughout the world studying traditional pharmacology and has presented more thorough information about holistic health and medicine than most allopathic researchers.

2.4 Delirium

Delirium is swelling of the membranes of the head, either from virus or other bacteria in the brain. If the cause is imbalance of the blood humour, the person is happy or giddy. If it is due to biliousness, there is ill-temper and constant frowning. If due to phlegm humour imbalance, the person is perplexed and weak; if due to black bile, the person is manic and wild (this happens very rarely). Furthermore, if the cause is blood humour, the temperature is often quite high. The delirium caused by yellow or black bile will cause raving. In all forms, the senses are not sharp. Valerian root infusion as a tea is helpful to calm the person. Adjust the proper humour according to the signs. Cupping the lower legs is advised as well; also a massage of the legs to absorb gas.

2.5 False Delirium

Raving and talking nonsense sometimes happen without swelling of the brain membranes, as when the person is feverish.

This condition is called false delirium. Treatment is treating the cause, as false delirium does not occur alone. Check the other signs and refer to appropriate section.

2.6 Stiffness

This condition comes on suddenly, and the person becomes motionless. Black bile is the cause, bringing obstruction to the lower section of the brain. The person is senseless and should be given a hot suppository or enema of two teaspoons of lobelia in one quart of water. If the person cannot be roused, a few drops of tincture of lobelia taken orally will usually suffice to bring him to his senses. When the senses are restored, give a black bile purgative, hot drinks and food, and rub the back of the head with oil.

2.7 Heart Failure

The signs of this are similar to stiffness, but in addition to the person being motionless and senseless, there is no breathing. The person falls down like a dead body. A complete obstruction of the brain causes this. Rubbing the feet and hands, especially the left hand, at the juncture of the thumb and palm on the beefy part, should be done with great force. Cardiac massage should be begun, and an ambulance called. If it is caused by prevalence of blood, some must be let out. Otherwise, an enema and suppository should be given to take out phlegm. Vomiting is a good sign. If there is no breathing at all, and no pulse, recovery is improbable. The difference between a heart failure and a fatal condition is that in simple heart failure, you can see a reflection of yourself in the person's eyes but in a fatal condition, this is absent. In rural settings, with no help available, it is recommended that even though the person may look dead, he should not be buried for seventy hours, because cases of spontaneous recovery have been recorded. If a mirror held to the lips shows no frosting, the person has turned blue, and the stomach is swollen, death is certain.

2.8 Lethargy

This is like a very heavy, unnatural sleep. Its cause is the prevalence of moisture in the brain, brought on either by phlegm or by blood. The remedy is to adjust the humour and use an enema. Make the person smell vinegar and feed him only light, easily digested foods. Another cause of lethargy is stomach gas. Clean the stomach by making this mixture: fennel seed, crushed, 5 grams; powdered ginger, 5 grams; and enough honey to make into a thick paste. Take one teaspoon with tea at each meal. Follow with a chickory-root enema. Put coriander as a spice in as many meals as possible.

2.9 Sleeplessness

The cause of sleeplessness is prevalence of dryness in the brain. It can come from imbalance of black or yellow bile or phlegm humour. Give an enema. Don't allow vinegar vapor to be inhaled, and avoid vinegar in foods, for it will increase sleeplessness. Put common dill under the pillow before sleep. Sweet basil in rose water can be smelled, too. Valerian root tea, or two 00 capsules of the same are very effective.

2.10 Lethargy and Sleeplessness

This combination of conditions is caused by a kind of brain swelling due to biliousness and phlegm, according to most healers. The signs are lengthy sleep, tiredness, or sometimes inability to sleep at all. If it is caused by swelling of the brain, the person will be wide-eyed and talking nonsense. The remedy is to combine the formulas given in sections 2.8 and 2.9 for the single signs of lethargy and sleeplessness. If there is much phlegm, use hot herbs; if biliousness is prevalent, give cold herbs.

2.11 Nightmares

The person imagines during sleep that some heavy object has fallen on him, or someone is chasing him, or some catastrophe is occurring. Therefore, shortness of breath is felt, and often a change in the tone of the voice. Cupping the legs, light eating before retiring, and enemas are all recommended.

2.12   Epilepsy

The person falls down completely senseless and has seizures, causing the limbs to assume contorted shapes. There is much restlessness and a feeling of heaviness in the head, and the veins under the tongue turn a greenish hue. This occurs spontaneously from time to time; if frequent enough, it can be fatal. Sometimes with children, it will occur seven or eight times in one day and never return. Something soft but firm, like a piece of wood wrapped with cloth, should be inserted in the mouth to prevent self-injury from choking on the tongue. When the seizure is over, give an enema. Do not give fresh fruit or goat milk, but instead allow the person to smell aloe wood.

2.13   Epilepsy in Children

Sometimes called hydrocephalus, and even children's gas or colic when the attack is mild. Children should not be carried too much or kept excessively warm or cold. Most healers recommend that nursing mothers avoid sexual intercourse until the signs pass, as it is felt this spoils the mother's milk and affects the child's brain. If there is constipation in the child, use a suppository, as it has an immediate effect.

2.14   Melancholy

This is an imbalance that prevents a person from thinking soundly and often leads to acting foolish, excessive loving, or sometimes to libertinism and great vanity. It is caused by an imbalance of the phlegm humour. Use an enema at wake-up and bedtimes. Eat only soft foods. Sexual intercourse has a remarkable effect in removing melancholy.

2.15 Madness

There are several kinds of madness. If it comes with anger and annoyance, it is called *mania*. If it comes with laughing, teasing, and annoying others, it is called "dog's disease." If it comes with frowning and being afraid of people, it is called "chorea." Some say madness is a kind of advanced melancholy, but it is not, for one of the factors of true madness is the burning of unnatural (corrupted) phlegm. Burning of natural phlegm causes melancholy, not madness. Adjust for phlegm humour inharmony. Take mother's milk and pour over the person's head and into the nostrils. Rub the body with violet and almond oils, and take frequent warm baths.

2.16 Vertigo and Giddiness

When someone stands up or moves abruptly and a "darkness" comes over the eyes, it is called giddiness. When the person feels everything turning around him, it is called vertigo. The remedy is to take an emetic and vomit. The cause is either in the brain or in the stomach. In either case, vomiting corrects it. Give one teaspoon of lobelia tincture every ten minutes until the effect is achieved. Lemon juice, sandalwood tea, and pomegranate juice are helpful to avoid this condition. If there is frequent vertigo, do not let the person become cold, and give hot foods.

2.17 Forgetfulness

The cause of forgetfulness is an excess of phlegm and its effect on the brain. Hot temperature causes forgetfulness, too. Remedy: give a chickory-root enema. Small amounts of tea made of 3 grains each of frankincense, sugar, and ginger are useful. Avoid cold water.

2.18 Paralysis

In this imbalance, half of the body becomes senseless and motionless. The cause of this is usually an excess of moisture in the phlegm humour, but sometimes imbalance in the blood humour can also be the cause. The cause of paralysis is swelling of the nerve endings. (If only one limb is affected, it is called slackness.) Do not give strong foods or herbs for four days. A light soup with cumin and cinnamon is good. After the fourth day, give the formula that ripens phlegm. Beneficial foods are pea water, clove, cinnamon, and black pepper. The phlegm will ripen from the ninth to the fourteenth day, at which time a purgative for phlegm should be given. After this, use an enema and lubricate the body with cactus oil. If the temperature is high, lower it. Never give hot medicine.

It should be noted that this kind of paralysis is not the same as that caused by viral infection from poliomyelitis. The only known treatment for the latter is large doses of organic iodine, as reported by J. F. Edward, M.D., in *The Manitoba Medical Review* (Vol. 34, No. 6, June–July, 1954, pp. 337–339). NOTE: A young man in Arizona died from poliomyelitis in 1977, after contracting an active case from his three-month-old daughter, who had been given a vaccine for polio. While the origin of his case has not been conclusively proved, it is possible and probable that this was the cause. Since polio has been nearly eradicated in the United States through use of the vaccine, most physicians under forty years of age have never seen a case. Whenever there is total paralysis and swelling of the thyroid glands, polio may be suspected. There is an urgent need for medical assistance if this is the case.

2.19 Weakness of the Limbs

A feeling of numbness or loss of sensation in a limb can be caused by either blood or phlegm imbalance. Adjust the proper humour and fast moderately for several days.

2.20 Paralysis of the Face

This happens when a part of the face is weakened. The signs are displeasure of the senses (corrupted sense of smell and the like) and a lack of appetite. Convulsions may appear if there is a stretching of the skin of the forehead and cessation of saliva and dryness in the mouth.

If there are no convulsions, start treatment four to seven days after the signs appear in the face. Eliminate as much food and as many liquids as possible. Put the person in a dark room, with a mirror so he can see himself. Have the person chew on a bit of nutmeg. It is said that if the paralysis of the face persists for longer than three months, it cannot be reversed.

2.21 Convulsions

There are two kinds of convulsion: moist and dry. There is excretion of phlegm in moist convulsions, and the onset is sudden. Dry convulsions come on gradually and there is excessive vomiting, sleeplessness, and depression. There may be weight loss.

The preparation for moist convulsion is the same as for ripening of phlegm. For dry convulsion, mix equal parts of violet herb and almond oil and massage the body, and have the person gargle with mother's milk.

Convulsions can also be caused by stings of scorpion and other insects, by a wound to the head or other part of the body, and by intestinal worms. Fight the poison, cure the wound, or expel the worm. In a city, any of these would be treated at a hospital emergency room facility or by a physician summoned to the scene.

Epilepsy can also cause convulsions, as discussed in 2.12. There is another kind of convulsion that occurs just after yawning and affects primarily the lower jaw and face. In this case, rub the body with warm flower oils.

2.22 Muscular Tension

There are so many sources of tension that it would be impossible to list them all in one book. The main cause of them all is that a nerve is pulled at from both sides, due to muscle spasm affecting a part of the body. The remedy is to discover where the spasm is located and apply constant direct pressure upon the place with the thumb and first three fingers bunched together. Apply steady pressure for twenty seconds, release for five seconds, and repeat until the spasm subsides. Follow with a massage with warm rose oil, accompanied by soothing music and a hot bath for ten minutes. Valerian root tea is specific for muscular tension.

2.23 Dystaxia

Dystaxia is the trembling of a limb. If the cause is phlegm, the signs are forgetfulness and the other signs of an imbalance of phlegm humour. The remedy is to use an enema. Excessive sexual intercourse can also cause spontaneous trembling of the legs and arms. If this is the case, drinking fresh goat's milk and rubbing the body with warm rose oil and eating lightly fried eggs are recommended.

2.24 Nictitation

This is the continuous trembling of a limb. The remedy is to warm salt and apply it as a plaster to the affected part. If it is not relieved, balance phlegm humour. Suppression of the menses can also cause this, in which case an emmenagogue is recommended (see 17.1).

2.25 Heaviness

In this condition, the person feels heavy all over and the eyelids may droop. The upper lids become red. There is frequent yawning and restlessness as before a fever, but no fever appears. The condition comes and goes. The preparation for balancing the blood and yellow bile humours should be given; allow some food even if the signs return. Chickory seeds with a little sugar are useful.

2.26 Nose Itching

The sign of this is itching in the nose but no pain. Give the person cold things to eat. The cause is found in biliousness, so give a biliousness purgative. If there is excess of blood, signaled by flushed face, nosebleed, or excessive heat, adjust the blood.

2.27 Eyebrow Pain

This is often caused by excess internal heat, in which case the pain commences at sunrise, along with fever, which continues until noon. It then gradually dies down until no sign is left throughout the night, but it starts up again in the morning. Dissolve 3 grains of camphor in flower oil and drop it in the nose, but do not inhale it into the nasal passages.

The Eye

General Considerations

To understand the function of the eye in terms of natural medicine, we must understand that it is the main receptacle of light in the body. It is related most closely with the lungs, as light is converted by plants into oxygen through photosynthesis, which is then breathed in by humans and other animals to sustain life. The direct rays of the sun, then, are the essence of life in that they are the pure form of oxygen.

Most often, little thought is given to how we use the eyes. First of all, we should endeavor to "see no evil," for if we accept that the mind originates much disease, looking upon harmful things is just like pouring sludge into the mind. Furthermore, at least once per day, one should rest the eyes. This is done by placing the palms of the hands tightly over the eyes, yet not so close as to cause much pressure. The object is to block out all light. Sit forward in a chair with the elbows on the knees, and rest the head in the palms of the hands. Remain in the position for twenty seconds, take the palms away for a few seconds, then repeat. Continue this for two minutes in the evening, to allow time for the eyes to regenerate their inherent strength.

As with all of the self-regulating organs, the eyes work nearly all the time without respite. The eyes are used in ways we are not aware of. For instance, in driving down the road, we pay attention to the many signs of traffic, looking out for other drivers, and so forth. But we also look at all of the many advertising signs, and things in the sky, and often over at other passengers. An advertising trade journal reported that the average person views 1200 such advertising messages each day! The mystics of the East sometimes seclude themselves for extended periods in darkness for the purpose of training the eyes to be under better control. We should all endeavor to have as much conscious control over what we look at as possible, for the same reason.

For the purposes of natural medicine, the eye is divided into parts consisting of seven layers, three moist vacuums and one hollow nerve, which is the receptacle for light. That portion which makes contact with the air and which can be touched is called the flesh layer and cornea. Under the cornea and flesh layer is the *original layer,* which is colored (in the normal eye, either blue or brown). In the middle of this is the "hole" that is the intake valve for light (*iris*). Behind the original layer is the *ball of moisture.* After the ball layer is the *spider layer.* After this, there is a layer called *solid moisture,* and finally the *crystalline layer.* After these layers there is the *retina,* then the *choroid coat,* and finally the *sclerotic coat.* These approximate the usual anatomical terms for the eye used in Western medicine, but we will use the terminology above in this section.

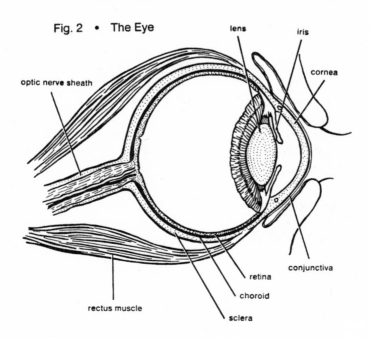

Fig. 2 • The Eye

lens

iris

cornea

optic nerve sheath

conjunctiva

retina

choroid

rectus muscle

sclera

Iridology

There has appeared in the past century a science of diagnosing states of health by looking at the eye, called iridology. Appendix I gives a chart showing the reflex correspondences of various organs in the eye, along with a brief discussion of the terminology and theory involved. A comprehensive study manual for iridology is Bernard Jensen's *Science and Practice of Iridology,* published by Dr. Jensen (D.C.), Route 1, Box 52, Escondido, California 92025. Some medical doctors and many alternative health practitioners use this tool as a guide for looking inside the body without using surgery. It cannot determine *what* is wrong but in most cases can tell *where* the problem is located and how far the condition has progressed.

3.1 Swelling of the Flesh Layer

If the cause is with the blood humour, the signs are that the eye is red, heavy, and painful and much secretion is noticed. If the cause is yellow bile, the signs are much burning and pain, but little or no secretion. With phlegm humour imbalance, the signs are swelling and a great quantity of excretion. If the cause is black bile, there is no swelling and no excretion, but the eyelids cannot close and touch each other and there is headache. If the cause is gas, there is no heaviness and no excretion. The remedy in each case is an enema and detoxification. Never drop any medicine into the eyes without consulting a physician first. Purgatives are advised for the appropriate humour, followed by bathing the eyes with mother's milk. Meat should be avoided, as should any boil-producing foods that are known to the person.

3.2 Appearance of Bloody Spot in Conjunctiva

Consult an eye specialist.

3.3 Pterygium

This is an inflammation of the wing or side of the bone of the nose, in line with the eye. Make a poultice of salt and apply to the affected place several times a day. Avoid phlegm-producing foods. A skilled physician should be consulted as soon as possible.

3.4   White Spot in the Black Part

A white dot appearing in the black part, or diaphragm, of the eye should be treated by washing with sea water (an infusion of nigari is an acceptable substitute). Using this procedure several times should remove the spot. If it remains, the brain needs to be cleared by taking a chickory-root enema for that purpose.

3.5   Swelling and Redness of Veins

If the eyes are red and swollen and there is copious tearing, and even the eyelids are wet, it is called *wet pannus*. If there is no wetness, it is called *dry pannus*. In both cases, relieve by enema. If there is only very slight redness of the veins, use the "golden suppository" composed of tumeric, 3 parts, and juice of aloe vera and rainwater, one-half part each in a cacao base. Take a tub bath before and after application to the eyes. If there is swelling accompanying the redness, do not eat hot foods or herbs—use cold ones.

3.6   Conjunctivitis

The difference between swelling and conjunctivitis is that the nature of swelling affects the whole eye (due to excess fluid and the like) while conjunctivitis affects the parts of the eye or skin. Conjunctivitis can be caused by gas, in which case the inflammation comes on suddenly. First a burning is felt on the corner of the eye, like the burning one feels when bitten by a mosquito or a fly. If the cause is phlegm, the onset is more gradual, and there is little or no pain. The remedy is to use a phlegm purgative. If the cause is gas, nothing is necessary, as it will disappear by itself after three or four days.

3.7 Itching of Conjunctivitis

This happens with conjunctivitis when the eyelids become red and sore. Salty and hot foods should be avoided. In addition to a phlegm purgative, if indicated, the eyelids should be rubbed very lightly with arnicated oil and the face and eyes washed every hour or so with warm water.

3.8 Hard Boil (Sty) in the Corner of the Eye

Such knobby boils sometimes appear in the corner of the eye. Their removal can be assisted by using a phlegm purgative, and as it softens, apply rose water as a wash.

3.9 Excessive Tearing

Excretion of tears is a normal bodily function, to remove foreign objects as well as an expression of human emotion of sadness or exalted joy. It is also the means to expel various superfluities that accumulate internally. What is spoken of here is tearing when none of the above causes is present. It is usually caused by overheating of the body, which can be corrected by rubbing with collyrium. If the cause is coldness, use lobelia infusion as an eyewash. It is sometimes also caused by weakness of the eye muscles. In this case, use exercises to strengthen the muscles. If there is unexplained tearing which stops after a few moments, it means that superfluities are trying to escape. Use a purgative and lobelia infusion.

3.10 Burning of the Eyes

A burning sensation in the eyes is also caused by excess heat of a part or organ of the body. Use a purgative. Pound fresh chickory, add safflower oil to it, and use as an ointment on the eyes.

3.11 Foreign Object in the Eye

If there is something in the eye, never rub it; it may be forced into and damage the eye. The best procedure is to wash the eye with warm water and pour mother's milk in as an eyewash. If the object that has fallen into the eye can be seen, use a piece of cotton twirled into a point to capture it. If it is an insect stuck in the eye, remove in the same way. If there is glass or metal or any object that cannot be identified in the eye, go to a doctor for removal with instruments appropriate for this purpose. When the object is removed, pour in mother's milk and add some white of egg to help soothe any damage.

3.12   Injuries to the Eye by Force

When the eye is hit by something and becomes swollen and red, the remedy is to boil fresh fruits, like apricot, plum, or tamarind together for fifteen minutes, and leave overnight, then filter in the morning and give to the injured person. Cup behind the head on the side of the injured eye. Afterward use a purgative, and put an ointment made of whole shirred egg and rose oil on the eye. This should remove the pain. If bruising is present, put egg yolk with coriander on the eye to try and speed recovery. Following any injury to the eye, an examination should be made to make certain that undetected damage has not occurred.

3.13   Ulcer of the Eye

An ulcer may appear on any layer of the eye. The least dangerous place is in the conjunctiva. Conjunctiva and cornea ulcers can be seen. Other ulcers occurring in the deeper layers cannot be seen, but cause severe pain. In time they may grow through the various layers and appear on the surface layer. Cupping should be applied behind the affected eye at the beginning of each week. If there is pain, a few drops of mother's milk will soothe. The ulcer must "ripen" to heal. Wash it with rose water to hasten the ripening, and afterward mix mother's milk with honey and apply as a salve.

3.14   Heaviness of Eyelid

This can be caused by gas, which is known by a feeling of sand in the eyes after waking up. Wash with juice of fenugreek. If this doesn't work, do not rub the eyes too much as they may be injured. If there is no relief, apply the phlegm purgative for conjunctivitis as given in Section 3.6.

3.15 Nyctalopia (Night Blindness)

The inability to see after sunset is often caused by prolonged exposure to a strong bright light. Apply honey with water of anise seed to the eyes. If it is severe, use a purgative.

3.16 Hemeralopia (Day Blindness)

The cause of day blindness is uncertain. Effective diet includes leg of lamb, beef brains, and unleavened bread. Massage the scalp with mother's milk and wash the eyes with cold water.

3.17 Eye Ache

A person feels a kind of beating deep in the eye that may extend outward toward the temples, and there is a slight prickling sensation. The pain is intermittent. Massage between the eye and the ear to stop this sensation from happening.

3.18 Bulging Eyes

Protection of the eyes without swelling can be relieved by taking an enema, using a purgative, and applying mashed dates over the eye as a salve. The diet should be restricted to smaller quantities of food until the eyes return to normal.

3.19 Projection of Cornea

This is caused by imbalance of both the phlegm and bile systems, so adjust for these both. Wash the eyes with warm water.

3.20 Ulcers of the Cornea

Since the cornea has four layers, ulcers may sometimes appear in any of them, sometimes in all. The remedy is to use purgatives and follow with the frankincense suppository.

3.21 Double Vision or Diplopia

If a person is born with this affliction, it usually cannot be cured. If it develops in childhood or later on, the causes may be epilepsy, sleeping on one side of the head, or extreme fright by loud noises. For children, it is recommended to hang down some bright red object on alternating sides of the head. In the case of the elderly, the cause is excess dryness. Dryness is always a sign of hot ailments, and the remedy is to consume a fruit diet and mother's milk. If the cause is slackness of the muscles of the eyeball, exercises must be done to strengthen them.

3.22 Dilation of the Eyes

Dilation is widening of the pupil, whether of the hollow nerve itself or the pupil. Another condition, called spreading, is the scattering of light in various parts of the eye, which is definitely a trouble of the nerve, not the pupil. When there is a widening of the hollow nerve, the pupil will usually widen, giving the impression of a dilated pupil. This is difficult to remedy, but mere widening of the pupil aperture can be cured, depending on the cause. A blow to the head should be treated the same as any injury to the eye. Excess phlegm can also cause dilation, in which case, use a chickory-root enema. If it is due to excess wetness in the eyeball, which happens mostly with boys, or swelling of the flesh layer, use a purgative. If the cause is dryness of the eye, the eye muscles must be strengthened the same as for poor vision.

3.23 Tightness of the Pupil

If the pupil contracts for no functional reason, the cause must be determined; it can be from excess wetness or dryness or a defect of the eyeball. Wetness and dryness can both be observed. A defect of the eyeball is apparent when there is an actual reduction in its size. The remedy for wetness and dryness is to massage the scalp with mother's milk and drop olive oil into each nostril (3 drops each side). If there is an excess of wetness, a purgative should be taken.

3.24 Imaginary Visions

This means the imagination of forms and figures, mosquitoes, and insects, and such. There are three stages to this problem. The first stage is prior to tears coming from the eyes. The second is appearance of stomach gas and wetness of the eye. The third stage is sharpness of the sense of vision. The clue to the onset of this condition is the appearance of more and more tearing in the eyes each day. When the imaginary visions become excessive, the stage of stomach gas has arrived. The clue that corruption of the layers and wetness of the eye has occurred is that the iris takes on different colors. The appearance of the third stage is accompanied by loss of health of vision and mind. This is not, in fact, a disease, as the vision actually becomes sharper as the stages progress. The person may actually "see" particles of gas ascending from his stomach and being scattered in the air. Because the person sees things that are not supposed to be there, he becomes totally confused. Sheep's brain and leg of lamb are recommended, along with detoxification of the system.

3.25 Glaucoma

This is a kind of wetness that enters from above in the head, suddenly or gradually, and stops in the pupil of the eye, and over time completely obscures vision. When the wetness thickens in the eye, it completely fills the hole for vision, and blindness occurs. If the wetness is thin, there may be some vision for color or form. The sign that it is glaucoma is that the pupil actually changes and vision is corrupted.

The only remedy mentioned for this involves cauterization, and since there are few practitioners of this, it would be difficult to locate a physician competent to perform such surgical procedure. The remedy given is reproduced here for general interest.

The remedy is to cauterize the temple on the side of the affected eye as soon as the signs of moisture appear in the pupil. It should be a deep cauterization, which should be dressed for three days with spinal cord of freshly slain sheep.

Then the site should be covered with a sterile cloth soaked with sesame-seed oil. Hard-to-digest foods and sexual intercourse should be avoided.

It should be known that there are several kinds of glaucoma, called cloudy, blue, glassy, green, white, yellow and red, gold, black, and scattered lightly. None of these is recoverable with natural medicine, except the white kind.

Western medicine has, to my knowledge, no *cure* for glaucoma, although there are drugs which can arrest its development if discovered and treated soon enough. My judgment is that Western medicine would be the treatment of choice in glaucoma. Wetness and overheating of the eyes occurs more in black, brown, and dark eyes, thus there is more glaucoma in persons with dark eyes.

3.26 Change in Eye Color

According to the science of iridology, there are only two true eye colors at birth, blue and brown. The eye contains delicate and sensitive nerves that pick up changes occurring in the body and reflect these in the eye. Drugs taken but not eliminated can cause a golden-brownish discoloration. The eye must be checked under magnification to see what the normal eye color actually is. (See Appendix I.)

3.27 Poor Vision

The cause may be excess of blood or phlegm. For excess of blood, balance the blood humour and take a purgative. Use eyebright as an eyewash. For phlegm, use a phlegm purgative and apply kohl (antimony sulfate) to the eyelids. Poor vision can also result from lack of natural heat, a usual condition of declining age. There is no cure for this circumstance, but kohl may be used on the eyelids.

3.28 Loss of Sight after Extended Darkness

If the cause is sudden emergence from a dark place, cover the eyes with a blue veil and avoid looking at sunshine until the eyes regain their ability to function normally.

3.29 Weak Day Sight

A few people are born with ultrasensitive eyes and cannot look at light. They usually cannot be cured of this condition, and must adjust to it by wearing sunglasses. Rubbing the eyes with smoke from ignited oil of violets is recommended to strengthen the eyelids and eye.

3.30 Snow Blindness

This is caused by looking at sun reflected upon snow for too long a time. The remedy is to hang black purslane from the person's neck and have him cast down his eyes at it. In addition, the room where he stays should have dark or very subdued light, dark carpets, and so forth. Pour mother's milk in the person's eyes. It is also very effective to put pounded bitter almond or apricot kernels on the eyelids as a poultice.

3.31 Feeling of Sand in the Eyes upon Waking

Though this feeling will go away on its own, the eyes should be cleaned with warm water, followed by a shower or warm bath. See also 3.14.

3.32 Slackness of Eyelids

Clean the eyelids with warm water, then apply juice of aloe vera as a salve. If the problem persists, the only remedy is corrective plastic surgery.

3.33 Eyelids Sticking Together

This occurs sometimes when there is excessive excretion from the eyes, as during allergy seasons. Pull the eyelids apart carefully, using warm water to help dissolve the mucus. If they have stuck to the eyeball, use great care in pulling the eyelids away and separating them. After that, take a half teaspoon of cumin and half a teaspoon of salt in half a cup of water; soak a ball of cotton in this solution and apply to the eyes for ten minutes. At night, rub rose oil on the lids.

3.34 Excess Skin Flap Growing on Eyelid

When small bits of skin appear spontaneously, the eyelids may actually thicken. It causes the eyes to be wet all the time from the excess weight bearing upon the eyeball surface. Use purgatives and dress the eye as in 3.33. If this does no good, go on a detoxification diet.

3.35 Growth of Extra Eyelashes

There is no particular danger from excess eyelash growth. They can be plucked out. To help keep them from turning in and irritating the eye, make the lashes straight and firm with honey to keep them from pricking the eye. A physician can probably cauterize the roots of a few excess hairs to stop them from growing back as a last resort.

3.36 Shedding of Eyelashes

The cause is usually food putrefying in the stomach. Use a stomach purgative to take out excess phlegm, which is sure to be present. A fruit diet is recommended until the shedding stops. The cause may also be a lack of nutrients reaching the area, in which case foods rich in niacin along with rigorous exercise should be the program.

3.37 Whitening of Eyelashes

Use a purgative and afterward take leaves of tulips, bruise them in olive oil, and apply to lashes.

3.38 Mange of Eyelids

Only diet will help here. Use a purgative first, then employ detoxification diet, emphasizing foods of a cold nature.

3.39 Excessive Perspiration of Eyelids

The pores of the eyelid need to be opened. Make them soft with olive oil, then use eyebright eyewash.

3.40 Hardening of the Eyelids

This is caused by excess bile, which causes difficulty in opening and closing the lids. Use the biliousness purgative and keep the eyelids soft with olive oil.

3.41 Swelling of the Eye

Swellings of the eye which are not due to any of the foregoing may respond to fruit-juice diet. Along with this, soak a few leaves of sumac in a half pint of rose water and use as eye drops during the day. At night, prepare a salve of purslane and chickory with rose oil.

3.42 Ulcers of Eyelids

Boil the skin of a large pomegranate along with the inner skins from about two dozen pistachio nuts, and add to half a cup of lentils that have been soaked in vinegar for several hours. Make a salve of this and apply to the eye until the ulcer subsides. Then put yolk of egg with a grain of saffron on the ulcer.

3.43 Swelling of Eyelids

The eyelids alone will swell when there is weakness of the intestine. The cause is almost invariably excess of phlegm, so use a phlegm purgative, follow with the detoxification diet, and use colonic irrigation if needed.

3.44 Boil on the Eyelid

Balance the bile humour. Apply Betonite (a diatomaceous earth preparation sold in most health food stores) to the affected area.

3.45 Dandruff of the Eyelids

Use a phlegm humour balancer. If it is chronic, scratch the area with a piece of hardened turbinado sugar until it is slightly raw, then apply collyrium.

3.46 *Ulcer in the Inner Corner of Eye*

For these ulcers, called sties, treat the body with a purgative first. Then, clean the ulcerated part with a piece of clean cotton and take away all pus. Keep it clean and it will go away by itself. If the tear duct is infected and blocked, clean the eye as above, then use eyebright wash, followed by a few drops of mother's milk to which a grain of finely ground saffron has been added. Put this on the ulcer to open it.

3.47 *Itching of Eyelids or Duct without Boils*

Use a systemic purgative, and afterward apply half a gram of pounded chickory with rose oil to the site of irritation.

The Ear

General Considerations

The sense of hearing is above all the other senses, as sound is connected with memory, the intellect, knowledge, and the higher faculties. For example, music is heard by the ears and affects the sense of hearing in a way that can produce an aesthetic sensation or even religious feelings. The trained mystics of the East work in practical ways with sound. The long sound of the vowel *a* (as in *father*) is often intoned in all of the esoteric schools to stimulate the heart center. The vibratory level of the sound *ah* has the ability to move the heart and mind in ways that other senses cannot perceive. All of the prophetic books have first been recited as poetry, and the faculty of hearing is necessary to respond to this. According to the science of breath, the vibratory level of the letter *a* radiates a *feeling* of sympathy, power, and magnetism. Likewise, the vowel sound of a long *e* gives a clear sound and feeling, like diving deep into the recesses of one's own soul. Physiologically, the *a* vibrates in the heart; the *e* vibrates up the nasal septum and stimulates the root of the pineal body, an organ of uncertain function that is admitted to have some relation to a vestigial homologue of a "third eye," a light-sensitive organ.

Figure 3 gives the basic anatomy of the ear. Generally speaking, little goes wrong with the ear, but when something does disturb the delicate inner mechanisms, the cure is difficult.

4.1 Earache

Earache due to swelling or ulcer is explained in 4.2 and 4.3. Other causes are from hot or cold temperament, which should be balanced with a purgative. Water retained in the ear after swimming or bathing can cause earache. Remove the water by jumping on one foot, on the side of the ache. A small piece of sterile sponge or cotton can be made into a wick and gently inserted into the ear opening to absorb the water. If there still remains water in the ear, take a piece of anise wood 20 cm long and bind a piece of cotton to one end, soak it with oil, and ignite it with a match. Insert the other end a small distance into the ear and the water will be completely absorbed.

If there is a worm or insect in the ear, try blowing smoke into the ear, which will probably cause it to come out. If this doesn't work, you probably will have to go to a doctor and have the ear irrigated to remove the foreign object. If a doctor is unavailable, try boiling peach leaves, or bruise the juice out of the leaves when fresh and use this (or the juice of aloe vera or vinegar) to kill the insect, which can then be removed with a Q-tip.

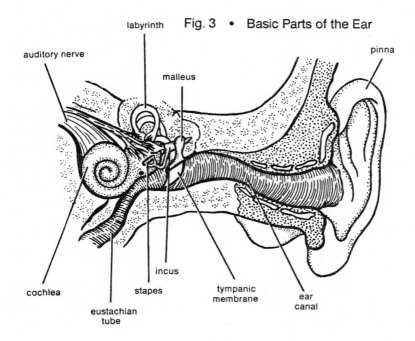

Fig. 3 • Basic Parts of the Ear

4.2 Swelling of the Ear

After first trying a purgative, examine the ear to determine if the swelling is coming from the inside or the outside. If it is swollen inside, there is severe pain, weakness of hearing sense, and often fever. Rub a composition of equal parts of sandalwood, magnesia and camphor, and coriander water inside and outside the ear, and pour a few drops of mother's milk into the ear to stop the pain. If this has no effect, drop linseed water into the ear to ripen the infection.

If the swelling is on the outside of the ear, there is obvious enlargement but usually no severe pain and no fever. If there is severe pain, soak hot cloths in a decoction of lobelia and apply as a compress. After two days, put this poultice on the ear: four large cabbage leaves boiled in pure butter; keep this on the swollen part for twelve hours and repeat if necessary.

4.3 Ulcer of the Ear

The signs are swelling and excretion of rheum. The remedy is to soak a wick with honey to clean the infection. Then mix honey, dragon's-blood, and frankincense in equal parts together and add half an ounce of rose oil; apply to the ear with a Q-tip.

4.4 Weakness of Hearing

Weakness of hearing, deafness, or lack of an orifice should all be treated with purgatives. The cause can be hereditary or due to old age. These cannot be helped by herbs, so the person with them is advised to consult a hearing specialist to see if a mechanical hearing aid will help.

4.5 Entrance of Stones and Similar Objects into the Ear

Remedy: Drop three drops of olive oil into the ear and have the person sniff black pepper to cause sneezing. When the person is about to sneeze, block the nose and mouth completely, and force the ear to expel the object. If this is not effective, seek medical help.

4.6 Ringing in the Ear (Tinnitus)

This trouble has psychic origins and often comes upon people who are overly intellectual and very anxious. Detoxification of the system should be accomplished first, along with relaxation techniques. It is helpful for the person to take up pastimes unrelated to his intellectual pursuits. There is no certain herbal cure. It has been determined that those who suffer from a constant ringing in the ears continue to "hear" the sound even if the auditory nerve is severed. This gives some credence to the view that there are auditory signals that are constantly going on but are normally beyond the range of our hearing. Many people have temporary ringing or buzzing of some kind in their ears. It is not understood by medicine why this occurs, but in the view of natural medicine, it is a sign and tone from another, higher dimension that needs to be heard. It can also be a temporary reaction to a blow or a very loud noise.

4.7 Bleeding of the Ear

The cause can be from a befouled stomach or from injury. In the former case use a stomachic, and in the latter case apply first aid. If the bleeding will not stop, boil a quarter of an ounce of gallnut in four ounces of vinegar and put a few drops in the ear, which should stop the flow of blood. If there is spontaneous bleeding from the ear from no apparent cause, it may be that the body is eliminating toxic blood or excess blood pressure in the brain. This condition will regulate itself. If the bleeding is due to the bite of a snake, consult the section on snakebite (see 21.27).

4.8 Cracks in the Ear

This mostly happens with children. Apply cupping between the shoulder blades and under the ear on the side of the injury. Wash the ear with mother's milk and apply sweet almond oil.

4.9   Itching of the Ear

Remedy: Boil a quarter of an ounce of wormwood in three ounces of vinegar; add ten drops of bitter almond oil to it and put a few drops in the ear.

4.10   Injuries Caused by Extremely Loud Noise

Strengthen the brain with a diet rich in greens, keep sweet scents about all the time, and burn rose incense.

Section 5

The Nose

General Considerations

According to natural medicine, the nose has two outlets, one going to the brain and the other to the throat and then on to the lungs. In yoga and other mystical disciplines, there are practices that involve breathing through alternate nostrils in order to balance both the brain and the lungs.

Relatively few ailments, apart from injuries, affect the nose. The hairs that grow in the nose gather minute particles and keep them from entering the head or lungs. The sense of smell is necessary for proper appetite and to perceive certain danger signals in the environment. Afflictions of the nose are often accompanied by troubles in another part of the head or face—thus specialists treat the group of "eye, ear, nose, and throat" diseases.

5.1 Corruption of the Sense of Smell

There are three kinds: (1) that a person perceives all scents as the same; (2) that different smells are perceived from the same scent; and (3) that some scents are perceived but others are not. In the last case, sometimes only sweet smells are noticed, or only sour scents. The remedy is to detoxify the brain by diet. If the person smells everything as foul odor, drop a few drops of musk oil into the nose.

A New York physician recently published information that

the complete corruption of the sense of smell is due to a zinc deficiency: he used massive doses of zinc to cure several drastic cases.[1]

5.2   Hemorrhoids of the Nose

An extra piece of flesh growing in the nose can be relieved by cupping the back of the head and using a purgative. A salve of common soda plant and myrrh is recommended as a nasal suppository. If this does not bring relief, surgical removal of the skin piece is necessary if there is obstruction of breathing.

5.3   Boils in the Nose

Remedy: use a purgative. If the boil is hard, soften with wax and oil.

[1] Arthur Berton Roueché, "Annals of Medicine (Disorders of Taste)," *New Yorker*, September 12, 1977, pp. 97–117.

Fig. 4   •   The Nose

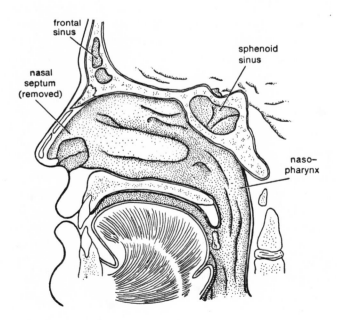

frontal sinus

sphenoid sinus

nasal septum (removed)

naso-pharynx

5.4 Ulcers of the Nose

If the ulcer is wet and draining, apply cupping to the sides of the nose and use a purgative. Afterward, rub with rose oil. If the ulcer is dry, rub it with wax and oil.

5.5 Nosebleed

There are many causes of nosebleed, some of which are discussed in other sections as a sign of another ailment. Check these sections in the index, especially if there are other signs present such as fever, vomiting, diarrhea, and the like.

A nosebleed can be controlled by binding the arms, thighs, and ears tightly and cupping the back of the head. If blood is coming out of the right nostril only, also apply cupping to the area of the liver. Apply cupping over the spleen if there is blood coming out of the left nostril only. The blood should be thickened after bleeding, which can be done with a diet of rice and lemon juice. In some mental diseases, blood must escape from the head, and does so through this mechanism. If the bleeding does not stop on its own, consult a physician.

5.6 Foul Odor Coming from the Nose

The cause may be a boil or ulcer, which must be treated first. If the bad odor is from phlegm, it may mean that the brain is infected. It may also be from gas rising from a foul stomach. In either case, purge the brain or stomach. Gargle afterward with oxymel and mustard seeds soaked in water for an hour, then strained. Dropping sweet-smelling oils in the nose is also recommended.

5.7 Bruising of the Nose

If there is an injury followed by blood and rheum, immediately try to put the nose back in its correct placement, as it may have been broken, and this will prevent a wrong mending that could obstruct breathing. Then make a paste of aloe vera juice, false acacia, and myrrh (equal parts) on a clean sheet of paper and paste this over the nose.

5.8   Excessive Sneezing

The usual cause of this is thought to be allergy. Sensitivity to substances can often be minimized by eliminating intake of all sugar, including the sugars of fruit, along with a general detoxification program. For intermittent irritation that causes frequent sneezing, drop rose oil into the nose and rub the same oil over the hands, feet, eyelids, ears, and on the top of the palate in the mouth. Mild sneezing is a sign of healthy reflexes; anything in excess is a bad sign.

5.9   Dryness of the Nose

The nose can become overly dry in the heat of summer. Eat humorally cold foods and beverages. A few drops of mother's milk will soothe and moisten the membranes.

5.10   Itching of the Nose

The nose often gets itchy in the colder months. Adjust the temperament for cold weather with a hot diet. If it seems to be the start of flu, take one 00 capsule of cayenne pepper and a half teaspoon of tincture of lobelia and go to bed under several heavy blankets. Repeat the dose every half hour until there is a profuse perspiration. After this perspiration breaks, sleep will follow and one will awake refreshed.

Section 6

The Mouth

6.1 Swelling of the Tongue

The remedy is to use a purgative and gargle. If the swelling has not passed away in three days, use syrup of lettuce seeds, chickory, and purslane in equal parts as a gargle. If this does not help, wash the tongue with linseed water first, then use a gargle composed of feverfew herb, white melilot, violet, and fresh seeds of cassia in equal parts, and add to one pint of pure water. In case of phlegmatic condition, mix some honey in with the formula; in the case of biliousness, mix some cooked figs

Fig. 5 • The Mouth

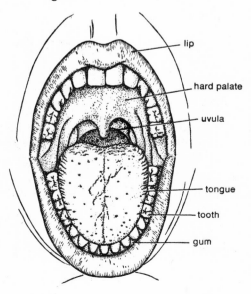

lip

hard palate

uvula

tongue

tooth

gum

in with it and add half an ounce of violet oil and three grains of purging cassia.

If the swelling becomes chronic, chewing on chickory and fresh coriander is recommended.

6.2 Heaviness of the Tongue

In this condition, the person has difficulty pronouncing words. If it is severe, the person cannot pronounce words at all. The cause is languor of the brain, which needs purging and detoxification regimen. If the cause is not languor of the brain but humoral imbalance, use the remedy for paralysis as found in 2.20. Cupping under the chin is sometimes helpful.

6.3 Enlargement of the Tongue

When the tongue becomes so large that it protrudes from the mouth, imbalance of the blood or phlegm humour is the cause. In the case of blood imbalance, balance the humour and rub sour pomegranate on the tongue. If it is a phlegm imbalance, adjust for phlegm and rub salt and vinegar on the tongue.

6.4 Slackness of the Tongue

The remedy is the same as for enlargement; see 6.3.

6.5 Split of the Tongue

If a taut, dry feeling exists in the brain, give the person plenty of fluids with a few drops of violet oil in each glass. Rub cucumber foam (obtained from rubbing two pieces of cucumber together) on the tongue. If the cause is stomach gas, it means that the digestion is off and a stomachic tea is needed. After cleansing the stomach, keep a few leaves of plum in the mouth.

6.6 Dryness of the Tongue

Lack of salivation is caused by excessive internal heat. Keep water of quince seeds and a little sugar handy and sip frequently.

If phlegm also comes on the coating of the tongue and there is further drying, rub oxymel on a piece of willow wood and put it in the mouth.

6.7 Burning Sensation on the Tongue

If this is due to eating a scalding substance, use a purgative, and eat very cold substances such as ice chips.

6.8 Itching of the Tongue

After using a purgative, gargle first with warm water, then with milk, then with sugar water, then with vinegar, then with rose oil. Grind dates and put on the tongue to soothe.

6.9 Growths under the Tongue

When something hard, like a gland, appears under the tongue, the cause is watery phlegm or blood. It must be surgically removed by a physician. Purge the phlegm humour.

6.10 Corruption of the Sense of Taste

This is a feeling of a bad taste in the mouth. The cause is prevalence of phlegm. Purge the phlegm and gargle with oxymel.

6.11 False Taste

False taste means that the person cannot taste at all. It sometimes happens that the general sense of temperature is also corrupted, and the tongue cannot distinguish between hot and cold. The cause is prevalence of moisture in the nerves of the tongue. After purging the brain, cook mustard seeds (half an ounce) with masterwort (imperial root, quarter ounce) in two cups of water. Cool and gargle.

6.12 Lesions of Skin of Tongue

Use a purgative and then boil equal parts of rose leaves, pomegranate flowers, and myrtle in two cups of vinegar and gargle.

6.13 Boils of the Mouth

Use a purgative and follow with a gargle made of vinegar in which coriander has been boiled for ten minutes. Add half a cup of Betonite when cool and gargle.

6.14 Other Mouth Sores

First use a general purgative. Then determine the basic imbalance of humour. If it is due to blood or black bile humour imbalance, gargle with a preparation of magnesia, pomegranate flower, and camphor. If the sore has a foul odor, gargle with vinegar and salt to remove the wetness and secretions. If the cause is phlegm, boil equal parts of celadine (a quarter to half an ounce), dates, and masterwort (imperial root) in a cup of vinegar and gargle. If the cause is bile, chew henna leaves or boil coriander with gallnut and pomegranate skins in vinegar and gargle.

6.15 Excessive Salivation

This can occur during sleep or at time of waking up. The cause may be excessive heat or moisture in the stomach. Purge the stomach by rubbing fresh chickory with a little salt and drinking it in water.

6.16 Bad Breath

If the cause is poor hygiene of the mouth parts, clean them with a teaspoon of salt in a glass of water. Gargle rose oil or sesame water in the morning. Endeavor to brush the teeth and clean the mouth three or four times a day.

6.17 Swelling of the Palate

The cause may be blood or phlegm humour. If the cause is blood, the appearance of the swelling is red and there is soreness. If the cause is phlegm, the appearance is white and there is no pain. Use proper purgative and gargle with the formula given in 6.14.

6.18 Whiteness of the Lips

Remove phlegm with detoxification regimen; afterward eat thick foods (breads, meat broths, and the like) and drop jasmine oil into the nose.

6.19 Cracks, Separation, and Dryness of Skin of Lips

Check the sections on mouth ailments to see if there are accompanying signs. Keep the lips covered with a pomade made of tragacanth gum (powdered), cooking starch, and powdered gallnut. Mix a little olive oil with it for consistency. Every pomade put on the lips should be covered with the skin that is inside an egg.

6.20 Trembling of the Lips

If the cause is excessive blood entering the veins of the lips, fasting should be commenced. If there is a great deal of stomach gas at the same time as the trembling, apply the remedy in 2.23. If the cause is in the brain, it can be a sign of the beginning of epilepsy or paralysis. Consult 2.12 and 2.18. Begin detoxification diet.

6.21 Shrinking of Lips

Stomach convulsions can cause this. Use a purgative and massage the body with warm oils.

6.22 Hemorrhoids of the Lips

The appearance of a projected piece of the lower lip from inside the mouth should be treated by purging the blood humour and the bile humour, followed by the pomade given in 6.19.

6.23 Swelling of the Lips

Adjust the phlegm humour and use pomade.

6.24 Boils on the Lips

Use a purgative and see 6.13 and 5.3.

6.25 Ulcers of the Lips

Apply pomades (see 6.19) and correct humour according to the signs.

6.26 Toothache

If the cause is eating excessively hot foods, swirl ice water in the mouth. If the cause is cold food, do the opposite.

Another cause is ill-temperament brought on by overheating of the body. In this case, gargle with vinegar and rose water. In the case of a cold temperament and lowered body temperature, gargle with water in which cooked brown rice has been soaked, and use a chickory-root enema.

Putrifying food in the stomach also causes toothache. Cleanse the stomach and use more coriander in cooking. If the cause is gas from improper digestion, gargle with cooked anise seed and cumin (about a teaspoon of each mixed together in a pint of pure water).

A toothache can usually be stopped quickly by putting one tablet of betaine hydrochloride on the offending tooth. If there are frequent toothaches, a visit to the dentist is in order, as well as a review of one's dietary patterns.

6.27 Dull Feeling of Teeth

Where there is a general ill-temperament along with the dullness, the cause is from excessive eating of very hard and sour foods. The remedy is chewing leaves of purslane, seeds included if possible. Eating warm lamb kabob or fresh warm bread is recommended. In the case of a cold intemperament, the preparation is apricot kernels mixed with the core of nutmeg, chewed well. If the cause is in the stomach, sour belching and sour taste in the mouth are the signs. Remedy: Purge the phlegm and bile humours and see a dentist regularly.

6.28   Decay, Cavities, and Worn Teeth

Purge the brain, using gallnut and masterwort (imperial root) in equal parts as a tea and see a dentist.

6.29   Accumulation of Tartar at Base of Teeth

The cause is the same as for general paralysis. Consult Section 2.20. The teeth should be cleaned regularly by a dentist.

6.30   Discoloration of Teeth

Yellowness of teeth is a sign of biliousness. Blackness is a sign of canker. In yellowness, clean teeth by rubbing with lentil flower and vinegar. In blackness, rub rose oil with powdered root of bramble bush on the teeth. With excessive whiteness of teeth, rub with mastic.

6.31   Loose Teeth

With children and the elderly, it is a natural condition, and nothing should be done. In others, the causes are prevalence of moisture in the system, hot blood, and decay of gums. A dentist is recommended for treatment to try and save the teeth. If one is not near a dentist and the tooth has to be removed, put pounded fresh fig leaves with syrup of green figs on the tooth for three days, and the tooth should come out quite easily. Afterward, consume much oranges and other citrus fruits.

6.32   Spaces between the Teeth

This occurs as normal variation of growth in some children. For cosmetic reasons, some people want such spaces to be corrected by orthodontic appliances, which can be quite expensive. If it happens in adults, the cause may be prevalence of blood, so use a blood humour purgative. If there is pain with the widening, it is prevalence of blood. If prevalence of phlegm is the cause, there is no pain. Give a phlegm humour balancer.

There is some normal stretching due to the wear of teeth as aging proceeds. This can be adjusted somewhat with special devices, for which a dentist must be consulted.

6.33 Itching of Teeth

A person cannot help gnashing the teeth. Take a purgative and avoid hot, salty, and sour foods. Gargle with vinegar, taking care not to swallow any sourness.

6.34 Gnashing of Teeth While Sleeping

Give a purgative for the brain, and massage the neck with oil before sleeping. (NOTE: To help children to grow teeth easily, rub butter, honey, and gum Arabic on the gums. Rub the roots of the gums with rose oil to help stop gnashing.)

6.35 Swelling of Gums

Use brain purgative and gargle with formula given in 6.28.

6.36 Bleeding Gums

The cause is usually poor nutrition or hygiene. Correct these factors, and help the gums back to health by rubbing with powdered lentil, magnesia, and gallnut in equal parts. Cold gargles are also helpful. A teaspoon of liquid chlorophyll as a mouthwash helps supply healing nutrients.

6.37 Ulcers of the Gums

If the gums are infected, it is called ulcer of the gum. After forty days, it is called unsound ulcer. Follow the advice given in 6.31 and balance the phlegm humour.

6.38 Diminishing and Receding of Gums

In children, receding of gums helps stimulate tooth growth. In other cases, use this formula: soak equal parts (about 4 grams each) of mashed dates, pomegranate flower, oak leaves, sumac leaves, masterwort, and carob bean in water for several hours. Mash soaked substances together and apply the pulp to the gums. Consume oranges and other citrus fruits in season.

6.39 Swelling of the Uvula

Remedy: Use a purgative and gargle. In case of presence of bloody discharge and biliousness, gargle with a preparation of equal parts of vinegar and rose water. In case of phlegm with the swelling, mix oxymel with mustard seed. In case of canker, use cassia in fresh cow's milk.

6.40 Slackness of Uvula

If blood humour is the cause, gargle vinegar and rose water and rub the throat with red flowers, sandalwood, pomegranate flower, and camphor. If it is caused by inharmony of phlegm humour, gargle honey water and use a purgative. In children, rub hard gallnut in vinegar and put on top of the child's head.

6.41 Diphtheria

This is a bacterially caused acute inflammation of the throat, which should be treated by a doctor, or at least tested to determine if this is the specific ailment. According to natural medicine, the remedy is to take a purgative and afterward gargle with sumac water and other humorally cold things such as boiled barley water. If there is no coughing, sour things can be given. If blood humour is the cause, cupping on the lower part of the legs is recommended. After about three days, the diphtheria will begin to ripen, at which time the person should gargle with sugar mixed with fresh goat's milk and warmed rose oil, to help eliminate the canker in the throat. After the canker sloughs off, gargle with cow's milk and honey to clean the rheum. Afterward, feed a dish of wheat bran, almond oil, and sugar.

If the cause of diphtheria is felt to be phlegm, use enemas and gargle radish juice and honey with a little vinegar; apply cupping to the back of the head and under the chin.

In the case of black bile imbalance, cup as for phlegm and

gargle cow's milk. Make a pomade of ground and sifted feverfew herb mixed with some narcissus and chicken fat for consistency, and apply to throat.

There is an intense kind of diphtheria in which the person is forced to open his mouth by spasms of the muscles, and the tongue hangs out like a dog. The cause of this is swelling of the throat muscles, which needs to be cured by enemas and treatment according to the trouble with the muscles.

In another kind of diphtheria, the person cannot talk and everything given as food comes out through the nose. If redness appears on the neck under the throat, it is a good sign. If difficulty in swallowing occurs, cup on the second vertebra on the back of the neck. If breathing becomes impossible, a tracheotomy is necessary. Treatment by a healing professional is suggested from the earliest stages.

6.42   Burning Hot Boils in the Throat, Gullet, and Trachea

The sign of gullet boils is severe pain in the gullet, especially when eating sour and hot foods. The sign of throat and trachea boils is feeling severe pain when talking and chewing. Remedy for all three kinds of boils is to drink fresh fruit juices but avoid cold water. Eat soft foods only. For throat boils, gargling with the medicines mentioned in diphtheria, such as sumac water or barley water, is advised.

6.43   Swallowed Needles

In the absence of medical aid, grind magnetic stone, such as iron ore, and drink one tablespoon with water in the morning. After a half hour, give a purgative. After the needle is emitted, try to strengthen the stomach (see Section 9, General Considerations, and 9.1 and 9.2).

6.44   Fishbone Stuck in the Throat

If it is possible to see the bone and remove it with a tweezers, do so. If not, have the person take in something slippery, such as seeds of mango. Make a fist and beat the person on the back between the shoulders to cause the bone to be expelled or to cause it to fall into the stomach, where it will probably be digested. If it is stuck halfway up or down, tie a whole dried fig on a string, let the person swallow it, and then draw it back out suddenly, to withdraw the bone. Another technique is to grasp the choking person from behind with a "bear hug" by reaching under his arms so that a fist can be made and held right in the solar plexus. Make the person bend over and, quickly and with force, pull up and backward to expel the object.

6.45 Narrowness of Food Passage

This can be determined if light things such as water and soup will not go down, but large hunks of food in mouthfuls are easy and painless. The remedy is to purge the phlegm humour. Also drink cooked anise seed, frankincense, mastic, and hyacinth, each a quarter ounce. Apply cupping under the chin.

6.46 Slackness of the Throat

Its sign is that there is difficulty in expelling breath through the throat. The remedy is the same as for narrowness of the throat, as given above in 6.45.

6.47 Itching of the Gullet

Remedy: Take a teaspoon of tincture of lobelia every ten minutes until vomiting occurs. Afterward, gargle with vinegar.

6.48 Vibration of Trachea

Vibration is a sign of convulsion, which often causes some hesitation and impediment to speech. The sign of vibration is often seen in the aged, whose speech may vibrate constantly. Gargling with honey and water is very useful.

6.49 Drowning

Use the techniques recommended by the Red Cross or other first aid for resuscitation. After the person has been revived, this regimen is prescribed: boil an ounce of cayenne pepper with an ounce of ground ginger in vinegar, filter, and pour in the mouth to arouse the senses. Then feed a dish of pea flour and milk to assist the lungs to work better.

6.50   Choking by Hanging

If the person is still breathing, free the neck and immediately check to see if there is foam in his mouth. If there isn't, immediately give an enema and massage the feet with ground mustard seeds. When the person has come to his senses, have him gargle with violet oil and warm water. (The *hakims* note that if there is foam in the mouth, there is no hope of reviving the person.)

6.51   Difficulty in Swallowing

This may be due to diphtheria or other signs mentioned in this section. If it is from bad temperament of the gullet itself, adjust the temperament according to the cause of humoral inharmony. Apply rose oil between the shoulder blades because the gullet is closer to the back than to the front.

6.52   Ulcers of the Gullet

The signs are pain in the gullet and extreme sensitivity to hot and sour foods, while oily foods alone can be eaten with no pain. Remedy: Take a small piece of white wax, put rose oil on it, and eat little by little. After this, drink honey water mixed with milk and sugar for two or three days, until the ulcer is gone.

6.53   Coarseness (Hoarseness) of Voice

The cause can be either catarrh or bad temperament. For catarrh, give syrup of marshmallow herb and gargle to stop the catarrh. Bad temperament needs a humour adjustment, according to the signs. The coarseness of the voice can be filtered by eating beans, dates, figs, almonds, sugar cane, honey water, or large raisins; each will smooth the voice.

The Chest and Lungs

General Considerations

Man can live without food for several weeks and without water for days, but without breath, life ceases after a few minutes. The lungs are the largest organ in the body, and we tend to think in terms of functions of the lungs rather than of the entire process of breathing.

According to natural medical philosophers, breath is not the lungs, as such or the air moved by them but a divine emanation of potentiality, carrying the essence of every human faculty at its beginning and making it manifest in the various physical organs as it circulates through the body.

It is assumed that God created the original breath of Creation out of the finer particles of the fire humour and created the hollow left side of the heart to serve as the storehouse and seat of manufacture of the breath in the body. The tissues and bones and all other parts of the body are also produced from the four humours; the breath is thus related to manifest matter.

From the heart, the breath passes throughout the body, pausing long enough at each part to convey the specific properties: the sense of sight to the moist crystalline lens of the eye, the sense of hearing from union with the auditory nerve, and so forth. While there is much to be said in relation to the theory of modern medicine that the mind originates all vegetative faculties, the only view of natural medicine is that the breath carries the divine vital essence of the faculty of an organ. It is interesting to note that the word *human* comes from two Sanskrit words, *hu* (divine) and *manas* (mind).

If an organ is missing, there then remains on the breath a vital potential that cannot be used up and so becomes superfluous, resulting in persistent ill-health, which seems to have no cure. Whenever an organ is surgically removed, the channels of breath are destroyed due to the severance of the nerve fibers and often of important ganglia. The circulating "divine mind" of breath, coming to an absent organ, is turned back upon itself, and there is a great sense of distress which nothing can relieve.

The breath thus relates very closely to temperament and emotional character. For example, moist intemperament occurs when the breath lingers overlong in any one of the phases of earth, air, or fire. An imbalance in the fire element would be characterized by a personality that is hot, impetuous, prone to anger, physically strong, courageous in danger, strong in desires, and so forth. The whole range of human emotional types can be worked out on this same scale of the breath in relation to the elements.

Inherent in the natural medical view is the idea that willpower should dominate the breath. Since breathing is a function of the automatic nervous system, we do not need to apply intelligence to continue breathing, although this should be done as a regular part of health maintenance.

A balanced breathing pattern is necessary for stable emotions and intelligent living. This is obvious when one takes the trouble to catch oneself in the midst of anger. The breath is always out of rhythm in anger, fear, or in any extreme emotional state. Application of willpower to the intake and expulsion of breath can open a whole new dimension of living. Mystics, yogis, and other Eastern people use exactly this principle to gain control over the lower kinds of appetitive actions—anger, fear, perverse desires, and so on.

The following is a simple and very beneficial exercise that requires no special training. It establishes a regular, rhythmic pattern of breathing, develops conscious control over an ordinarily unconscious function so that the higher levels of understanding come into play, cleanses the superfluous matters from the breath, and balances all four of the bodily humours:

Sit in a relaxed position with the eyes closed. When inhaling, draw breath into and inflate the abdomen first, then the chest. On exhalation, reverse this.

To balance the Earth element: Inhale through the nose, exhale through the nose, four times.

To balance the Water element: Inhale through the nose, exhale through the mouth, four times.

To balance the Air element: Inhale through the mouth, exhale through the nose, four times.

To balance the Fire element: Inhale through the mouth, exhale through the mouth, four times.

This exercise should be done every day, ideally at wake-up, one hour after each meal, and at sunset.

In the inhalation phase of the breath, the innate heat or vital force is built up, and on expulsion it is dispersed. Simultaneous with the expulsion of breath is the appearance of the phenomenon known as the aura or atmosphere (a sensation resembling a gentle current of air, sometimes perceived as a color, rising from the limbs or body to the head).

In addition to the exercise given above, there are in every community teachers of yoga and other disciplines who teach conscious control of the breath as a means to regulated health. Great profit can be had in this discipline alone.

The expelled breath is that which separates the superfluous matters from healthy matter. Thus, one who has poor breath also has poor internal health. Disease can also be explained from this doctrine, in that the cycle of the breath is not in harmony with the process of formation of the humours of the body. Presence of the signs of disease indicate an abnormal humoral state, either an unbalanced innate heat or a conflict between innate heat and the heat of foreign substances (such as bacterial decomposition).

Any change in rhythm of the breath will in itself cause loss of natural immunity to bacterial agents. Since there must be an outflow of superfluous matter, any holding back of isolated microorganisms in the tissues will allow them time to develop into active colonies. This leads to structural organic changes in the body, called symptoms of disease.

A rational explanation for certain "miraculous" cures can be found in cases where long-standing blockages of the circulation of the breath have been removed, either suddenly or gradually. Restoration of the normal flow is often enough to allow the body to rid itself of the accumulated superfluities and resultant symptoms.

It should be remembered that smoking, air pollution, and poor posture can all contribute to disease by disturbing the regulated flow of the breath.

7.1 Asthma

Asthma is a chronic affliction of the gullet, recurrent and difficult to cure. The sooner it is treated, the better. The signs are expulsion of phlegm when coughing, hoarseness in the chest, wheezing, difficulty in breathing, and rasp in the lungs—all signs that the cause is phlegm.

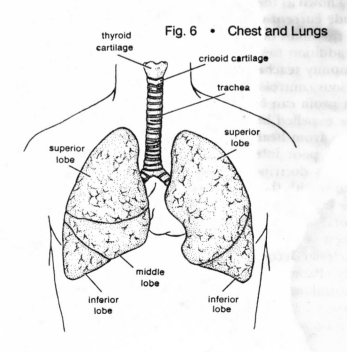

Fig. 6 • Chest and Lungs

thyroid cartilage

cricoid cartilage

trachea

superior lobe

superior lobe

middle lobe

inferior lobe

inferior lobe

The remedy is first to eliminate all foods that produce mucus such as milk, eggs, cheese, fruits, and all sugars of any kind. Foods high in iodine must be eaten, such as kelp, which also help replace minerals stripped out with the phlegm (consult the chapter on detoxification). Use purgatives, especially lobelia, and if vomiting is provoked, there is no harm. Coffee or chickory-root enemas should be employed whenever there is danger of an attack that could interrupt or stop breathing. They can be given every ten or fifteen minutes for up to two hours, if necessary, to keep the elimination of phlegm continuous.

Syrup of hyssop with warm water three times a day is recommended after a bout with asthma. White meat of turkey with plenty of spices is also recommended. When the phlegm seems to be building up, take garlic, with honey to soothe the throat if it is raw from coughing.

Dr. Edward Shook's preparation or remedy for asthma attacks and all afflictions of the lungs is one of the finest herbal remedies I have used. It is prepared as follows:

2 ounces slippery elm bark (powdered)
1 ounce horehound (cut)
1 ounce garden thyme (cut)
1 ounce red clover tops (cut)
1 ounce yerba santa
1 ounce lobelia inflata
1 ounce resin weed (leaves, cut)
1 dram capsicum (cayenne pepper)

Put all the above into two quarts of distilled water in which is dissolved an ounce of potassium phosphate (K_2HPO_4), if obtainable. Stir well and let stand for two hours. Cover tightly and simmer for thirty minutes. Strain, pressing out all liquid. Return to saucepan and reduce to one pint. Add twenty-four ounces of blackstrap molasses and eight ounces of glycerin. Bring to a boil and simmer five minutes very slowly. Cool and bottle. For spasmodic asthmas, the dose is one tablespoon every hour until relief is obtained. After this, take one tablespoon three or four times a day. For children, one teaspoon according to age; ages four and up, half the adult dose.

If there is pain, give about a quarter ounce of half-pounded linseed with honey, which should relieve the pain immediately. Rub the chest with linseed oil and beeswax.

There are several causes of asthma, according to the *hakims*. One is from *hot gas*, which is evidenced by these signs: thirst, hard beating of the pulse, and labored breathing, coming in hard gasps. For this, apply cupping on the left arm, give laxatives in beverages, and rub the sides.

Another cause given is *internal heat affecting the lungs*. The signs are hard beating of the pulse and thirst, but the breathing is not as labored. Remedy: Adjust with cold drinks and a cucumber pomade on the chest. Another cause is *slackness of the chest muscles*, which is evidenced by soft beating of the pulse and soft breathing. The muscles must be strengthened. Rub oil of narcissus on the chest and balance the humour as for paralysis in 2.20. Gargling with milk and cinnamon with honey added is also recommended.

If the cause of asthma is *excess dryness in the tissues*, the voice is changed to a somewhat higher pitch, and there may be thirst and a tendency to desire to drink liquor. Remedy: Give fruit juices and take sitting baths in water made from violet, cucumber, and marshmallow. Drink plenty of fresh milk.

If the cause is *cold nature of the lungs* (known from lack of thirst and soft pulse) give the person hot-natured foods. If the cause is *inflammation of the lungs*, a sense of lightness of the body, and coughing without phlegm are the signs. In this case, as with all others, use a coffee enema and adjust the proper humour. Put a pomade made of common dill and fennel seed on the chest.

Fullness of the stomach can also cause asthma. This can be corrected by coffee enemas, fasting, and improving the digestion.

Other causes are *swelling of the lungs, diaphragm, or liver*, which are discussed later.

7.2 Coughing

The signs and kinds of coughing remedies are as follows:

Blood humour   The signs are hard beating of the pulse, hot temperament of the breath, and redness of the face. All these are due to hot temperament of the liver. Drink cold-natured drinks.

Descending of superfluities from the brain   There is a tendency to sleep all the time, along with coughing. Gargle cooked marijuana seeds and keep a bit of gum Arabic in the mouth. A variation of this problem is that the substance coming down from the brain goes into the lungs and is thickened there. The signs are expulsion of phlegm while coughing, heaviness of the chest, runny nose, and congestion. This is treated with a drink of cooked fig, milk, and hyssop (equal parts). Keep some cayenne pepper with sugar and rose essence in the mouth.

Moisture of lungs and chest   A great deal of phlegm comes out when coughing, and the voice is hoarse. This happens mostly with the elderly and those who have moist temperament. Use the treatment given for asthma in 7.1.

Roughness of lungs from smoke or dust, or loud shouting   Remove the person from the smoke or dust or other cause. Moisten the lungs with syrups of barley and marshmallow (equal parts), dissolve in water with half an ounce each of sugar and almond oil added. Also, rub the navel with olive oil and the anus with butter.

Boils or ulcer of the lungs   The signs are fast beating of the pulse and a burning sensation on urination. Cold drinks make the person feel better. The remedy is to cup the chest and use purgatives.

Fullness of the stomach   Use an enema and limit intake of food.

Biliousness   If corrupted bile has reached the lungs, a blackish or dark-greenish substance comes out when coughing. Give boiled bran of wheat with sugar or honey, then adjust the bile humour.

Water or fluid entering the larynx The coughing will not stop unless the substance is thrown out. No treatment is advised. If there is so much congestion that it becomes difficult to breathe or swallow, the throat and chest should be rubbed with oil and an emetic is advised to clear the larynx and trachea so that function can be restored.

Cough powder This is a good remedy for cough to relieve general irritation of the throat and lungs:

Equal parts of (all powdered fine):

Skunk cabbage
Horehound
African cayenne
Bayberry bark
Valerian root
Gentian

Mix with three ounces of molasses and take a teaspoon with hot tea.

7.3 Blood Coming from the Mouth

The source of the blood must be determined. Blood can be coming from the parts of the mouth, from the head, or from the inner organs. What comes from the mouth parts is ejected with saliva. If it is coming from the head, it seems to come from the palate, and there may be light-headedness. If it is coming from the larynx and trachea, the blood is emitted when clearing the throat and comes out a little at a time. There is no coughing. Blood coming from the trachea is foamy, and there is coughing and pain.

There is also foamy blood if it is from the lungs, but there is coughing with or without pain. Blood coming from the chest is small in amount and is ejected with severe coughing. If the blood is coming from the stomach, spleen, or liver, it comes out by vomiting.

Remedies for each of these sources of bleeding are:

Parts of mouth:	Gargle cooked astringent things such as pomegranate flowers, gallnut, and myrtle.
Head:	Cup on the cephalic vein and gargle cooked astringent things such as pomegranate flowers, gallnut, and myrtle.
Larynx and trachea:	The above medicine, held in the mouth but not swallowed, should stop bleeding.
Lungs:	Apply cupping on the legs and adjust the temperament. If further measures are needed, put astringents on the chest, but only if the lungs are not swollen.
Chest:	Take the medicine as above and rub the chest. Chest ulcers often heal easily, due to the large supply of fresh oxygen in that part.
Stomach and other parts:	Consult appropriate section for specific body part.

In every case of bleeding, chewing purslane leaves or drinking a little syrup of purslane is recommended. If pressure of blood is felt in the lungs but there is no coughing, gargle vinegar and rose water and drink a few ounces, too. If there is coughing, mix ash of fig wood with water and sip this occasionally. Consult a physician as soon as possible.

7.4 Rheum Coming from the Mouth

This may be caused by the discharges of pneumonia, pleurisy, or tuberculosis (these are discussed in their own sections). If rheum is coming from the mouth parts or the larynx or throat, the cause may be diphtheria or other swellings. If rheum is coming from the chest, the remedy is to soften the phlegm. Make a pomade of beeswax, oil of fennel seed, and a little hen's fat and apply to chest. Never use astringents or cold foods. A drink made of cooked hyssop, fig, and licorice root is useful to open all swellings of the diaphragm and chest.

Substances from the chest entering the lungs are expelled via the trachea. There is no need to force it out.

7.5 Pleurisy

Pleurisy is swelling of the lungs. It is caused by imbalance of heat, whether of the blood, bile, or phlegm. The signs are high fever, severe asthma, heaviness of the chest, redness of the face and cheeks, and thirst. Apply cupping on the chest, then use a laxative or chickory-root enema.

If the pain and swelling are on the left side, the left cheek will be red, there will be a feeling of heaviness in the left side, and the person will prefer to lie on his left side. If the swelling is in the right lung, the opposite signs will be noticed; also in this case there will be some saliva running out of the mouth. If only one side is affected, the cupping should be done on that side.

After cupping on the appropriate side, put on a pomade made of equal parts of dry violet, linseed, goat's milk, barley flour, and common dill. Boil them all in water, with a little sesame oil mixed in, and apply lukewarm to the chest.

In chest afflictions, astringent medicines such as fennel or even cold water should never be given. To lower a fever, give nonastringent substances like cucumber juice, watermelon, and pumpkin juice. A fairly sweet mixture of vinegar and honey may also be given. If there is difficulty in breathing, give a coffee enema and laxatives and pour lukewarm water on the chest and sides to relieve pain.

7.6 Notes on Swelling

It should be known that swelling has three resolutions: (1) It ripens and comes out, (2) it jells, or (3) it becomes hard.

The sign of ripening is the gradual day-by-day diminishing of signs.

The sign of jelling, or turning to pus, is a worsening of the signs, especially as it begins to ripen. The fever and pain then go away, but heaviness is still felt in the chest. Then severe asthma and dry coughing, heaviness, and pain reappear. This kind of swelling, when ripened, will open and try to find its way out. Usually, blood alone or blood with a little unripened substance will first come out, followed by expulsion of the ripened phlegm. Pus usually "opens out" by means of reflexive actions, such as vomiting, severe anger, or a sudden movement. If, after ripening, it does not come out, it must be assisted.

If the swelling is hardening into phlegm, the signs are excess saliva, heaviness in the stomach, asthma, and absence of signs of heat. Make a pomade of mother's milk and soft wax and apply to the chest. If there is phlegm, the temperament must be adjusted for phlegm. When there is hardened phlegm, sometimes it beads into small stones, and then the coughing stops.

7.7 Tuberculosis

This is a lung ulcer. While it can be detected by regular chest x-rays, the active stage is known by the signs of hectic fever, and phlegm matter emitted in coughing. The matter ejected is some form of moisture. A natural test for tuberculosis is that the substance coughed up will sink in water and has a very foul odor when burned. While there is no immediate cure, the use of fresh air, sunshine, exercise, heat, light, rest, and similar aspects of nature cure are recommended. Avicenna said that a person affected with tuberculosis could live for twenty years, with proper care. Galen said that he cured every tuberculosis patient whose treatment had been initiated from practically the first day of signs.

If there is pain, apply cupping to the chest and give a soup of cooked barley with honey. Everything useful for hectic fever is useful in this case. Avicenna recommended giving rose conserve for tuberculosis, except to pregnant women.

7.8 Swelling of the Diaphragm or Internal Pleura

There are many names for vague symptoms of upper stomach pain; some call this pleurisy. True pleurisy, as described above, is a swelling of the pleura, or the membranes of the respiratory organs. Impure pleurisy, which is what is described here, is swelling of the muscles between the ribs, or the swelling of the membranes covering the back muscles. Diaphragmitis is a swelling of the membrane surrounding the stomach and the liver. There are other forms of swelling that affect the membrane between the digestive organs and respiratory organs, but there is no differentiation of these forms in treatment. In these cases of swelling, put a flower oil on the chest, or between the shoulders if the signs are coming from there. The difference between pneumonia and these swellings is that in pneumonia the pulse is erratic or "wavy" and there is severe asthma. In diaphragmitis, the person may become irrational.

Sometimes swelling of the liver is quite similar to pleurisy. The difference is that with swelling of the liver, the person's skin usually has a yellow color and there is no coughing; there is heaviness and pain in the liver, and the urine is very dense and concentrated in color.

Each of the above swellings will become ripened and should be treated before they turn into rheum. Give cabbage water, barley water with sugar, lots of butter and honey. Lying down on the affected side is helpful.

There is false pleurisy that can be mistaken for swelling. In this case, gas is imprisoned between the membranes around the sides and the person feels pain. Because the gas cannot escape, it appears almost like actual swelling of the membranes. The test for false pleurisy is that with simple gas, there is a lightness to the chest or other part, and also an absence of fever.

7.9   Rheum in the Chest

When swelling of the lungs ripens and the phlegm matter gathers and becomes thickened in the area around the lungs, it cannot be excreted by the lungs or in the urine. This is difficult to cure. Since the substance is not eliminated, hectic fever comes. To soften the substance and help eliminate it, give roots of fig, hyssop, plum, licorice, black raisins (in equal parts, ground together), and mix with almond oil and sugar to form little pills. Diuretics will also help. The substance may penetrate to the bladder or kidneys in an attempt to come out, and if this occurs, give any remedy that cleans the bladder and bowels, such as Betonite (a half cup daily).

7.10 Chest Pressure

The causes are exposure to extremely cold weather, cold wind, excess consumption of ice water, and smoking marijuana. The sign is lack of ability to expand and contract chest. Put warm rose oil or olive oil on the chest and drink warm milk with honey.

Section 8

The Heart

General Considerations

Heart disease is the leading cause of death among adults in America. There is a great deal of information and research about the causes of heart problems, much of which is focused upon diet and exercise. It is beyond the scope of this book to review all of the available literature on the subject of heart disease, but a few directions for keeping the heart healthy are in order.

The heart is the most important organ, and its treatment should always be commenced at the first sign of inharmony.

In the section on breath, it was explained that the heart is not just a muscle that pumps blood about the body. According to the great natural physicians, it has the further, even more important, function of acting as the storehouse and seat of manufacture of the breath.

Good exercise habits, then, are vital, for if the heart is not strong it may lead to stagnation of all inherent functions of the body. It is possible that "heart attacks" are nothing more (or less) than the atrophy of its capacity to generate the vital force of life itself. In the view of natural medicine, therefore, exercise is necessary not only to strengthen the heart but also for the health of all the bodily systems.

Obviously, one must map out a reasonable program of physical fitness in keeping with age, general level of health, season, and so forth. Dr. Sheldon Deal of Tucson, one of the prominent natural physicians in the Southwest, said that if one performed a simple set of exercises, it could be virtually *guaranteed* that one would never die of a circulatory congestion.

Here are his recommendations for keeping off the page of coronary statistics:

1. Begin with a thorough physical check-up to make sure there are no present medical problems.
2. Run in place, lifting the feet lightly, for one minute every other day for a week.
3. For the second week, extend the time to two minutes.
4. For each successive week, increase the time you run in place by one minute per week. After four weeks, run every day and increase the time until you are running five minutes each day.
5. After reaching five minutes, you can increase the tempo of the running and lift the legs higher, to promote more vigorous stimulation of the circulatory system.

Although it may not be possible to guarantee that someone won't die from heart attacks, this simple regimen, done each day, will certainly ensure that the all-important circulatory and respiratory systems are getting ample exercise.

Common sense dictates that smoking be eliminated and a healthy diet adopted, low in salt, meat, and animal fats. It is impossible to provide a single diet in this book for all people, because every person's needs and general state of health are different, but it is important to become conscious of what you eat, to begin to study and learn about the composition of foods and how the food affects the body. Many people advocate a salt-free diet, but the chlorides in salt are the only readily available source of manufacturing ingredients for hydrochloric acid in the stomach. This may explain why people use salt to excess: the body craves it to produce more hydrochloric acid to assist digestion of excessive amounts of food. Remembering the principle of natural medicine, "Fasting is the best medicine," it can safely be recommended for the average American that at least *less* food be consumed daily.

Not much information is given in the Eastern texts on natural medicine about heart disease per se, because it was so rare. In any agricultural society, the people eat simply and get plenty of exercise, so they do not have heart problems as we have them in the West. One man I knew from Badakhshan, Afghanistan, said he had never known anyone to die from a heart attack. In fact, he didn't even understand the concept very well!

8.1   *Heart Palpitation*

When palpitation becomes severe, it will be followed by fainting. There are three causes of palpitation: (1) the heart itself, (2) the stomach, brain, intestine, womb, lungs, or diaphragm: or (3) the total system, including the heart.

If the whole body is affected, the specific parts must be located and corrected. Check the index for sections which have palpitation as a sign of a specific ailment. If only the heart is affected, use a purgative and coffee enemas. Sometimes a person who has the "dry heaves" or excessive vomiting will have heart palpitation. Give spearmint tea as a stimulant, and energetic high-calorie foods.

Another cause for palpitation is living in an excessively warm climate. If one's temperament cannot take excessive heat, a change in climate is recommended.

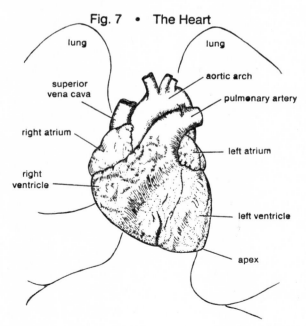

Fig. 7   •   The Heart

lung

lung

aortic arch

superior
vena cava

pulmonary artery

right atrium

left atrium

right
ventricle

left ventricle

apex

8.2 Fainting

If the causes of palpitation are not removed, fainting will result. When the cause of fainting is not corrected, it can lead to death. There are three kinds of fainting: (1) the soul is weakening; (2) the soul is congested; and (3) the soul lacks generative force. The causes of weakening of the soul are vomiting, extremes of happiness, overindulgences, and physical pain. The causes of congestion of the soul are excess of fullness (especially of drinks), sadness, great and sudden fear, or shock. The cause of lack of generative force is a bad temperament, or poor food, which cannot increase the potentiality of the soul. The long-term remedy in each case is to remove the cause and strengthen the soul and temperament by meditation, breathing practices, and religious contemplation. If the cause of fainting is excess of heat, give cold foods and energetic drinks like sandal tea after the patient is aroused. If the cause is cold, allow the person to smell hot vapors, such as musk. Adjust the temperament, in the case of heat, by pouring rose water and cold water on the chest. However, never pour cold substances on the chest if the cause of fainting is from stomach foulness. In this case, make a tea from one-half ounce of powdered ginger and one-half ounce of crushed fennel seed, mixed with honey for consistency. Give half a teaspoon before each meal to balance digestion. Once the stomach is cleansed, eat stewed chicken and meat broth and rub the chest with cabbage oil.

Other substances to substitute for the hot ones given above are: musk, saffron, ambergris, aloe wood, mint, cardamom, amber, camphor, magnesia, marshmallow, apple, and coriander.

If there is great perspiration when the person faints, it is because the pores are opening to allow toxic matters to escape. Excessive perspiration can be stopped to avoid dehydration by grinding leaves of myrtle, soaking in water, and rubbing this on the body.

In all cases of fainting except excess of perspiration, vomiting is recommended immediately after fainting. This can be effected by successive teaspoon doses of tincture of lobelia, every ten minutes until the result is achieved.

Strangulation of the womb can cause fainting (see 17.26).

A person who faints may have a slightly yellow color to the skin and a weak pulse. In a serious case of fainting, the person cannot open the eyes but will understand you if you call his name. If the person cannot understand or hear you, that is apoplexy, not simple fainting, and needs immediate medical help.

8.3   Swelling of the Heart

When the soul becomes weak because of long illness and this weakness reaches the heart, it causes swelling. It is said that this swelling is mostly of a cold nature, because if it were of a hot nature, it would cause death immediately. Of course, cold-nature swelling that reaches the heart can also be fatal, but if it reaches only to the outer surface or skin of the heart, it can be cured. If it is not cured, the person loses weight day by day until he dies. The sign is a feeling of heaviness in the chest close to the cardia. The person looks as though he may faint. There is heart pressure, the face is very yellow, and the eyes become excited. The remedy is to put cooked dates, white clover, and wheat bran on the chest and cardiac area. Give foods to strengthen the heart, such as beef heart, brewer's yeast, bone marrow, dairy products, egg yolk, green leafy vegetables, peas, beans, nuts, lemons, and oranges.

8.4   Odd Sensations in the Heart

The person may feel "smoke" inside the chest coming from the heart or other strange feelings. This can cause fainting and confusion. Give foods to moisten the temperament and use a purgative to balance the bile humour.

8.5   Heart Pressure

When pressure is felt, there may be fainting and saliva running out of the mouth, followed by hiccups. Give a coffee enema to take pressure off the liver, give a bile purgative, and use relaxation techniques of massage and soothing calmative drinks such as chamomile, valerian root, catnip, hops, and the like.

8.6 Heart Attack

The person feels senseless for a short time, but immediately comes back to his senses. There may be convulsions because of the pain, and thus perspiration. Obviously emergency medical aid should be summoned immediately. If there is none available, a coffee enema can relieve pressure on the internal organs; first aid for resuscitation should also be given if necessary. If the attack is not fatal and you are away from any medical aid at all, purge the bile humour and try to rebuild the heart with a strengthening diet as in 8.3, but eliminate the eggs and dairy products.

8.7 Sensation of the Heart Coming out of the Chest

This is caused by toxic matter in the blood and befouled yellow bile humour. Give bile humour purgative, rose water, willow water, and syrup of sandal.

8.8 Feeling the Heart Is Being Pulled Downward

This feeling is caused by phlegm reaching the area of the liver and surrounding it. The person may feel slight pain and appear to be ready to faint. Use a phlegm purgative.

8.9 Feeling of Fluid in Heart Area

The person feels that his heart is moving in water in a convulsive movement. The *hakims* say this is a kind of palpitation caused by excess moisture imprisoned under the skin of the heart. Make a salve of red flower blossoms, saffron, and hyacinth, mix with mint, and apply to chest. Fortunately or unfortunately, the best way to assimilate heart moisture is by feeling anger!

Sometimes the above-mentioned moisture becomes dried, yet remains inside because of unbalanced heat. The sign of this is that the heart doesn't expand, breathing becomes difficult, the strength dissipates, and anger appears. The remedy is to use laxatives and moistening pomades on the chest.

The Stomach

General Considerations

According to natural medicine, all illness originates in the stomach. It has been explained in earlier chapters that if the stomach is overburdened or is not functioning efficiently, there will eventually be damage to other organs of the body. Where the damage occurs depends on each individual's inherited constitution and other factors.

One of the first problems with digestion, usually due to excess food consumption over a long period of time, is insufficient hydrochloric-acid production. This deficiency can be determined from reading the iris, according to the science of iridology (see Appendix I).

The Five-Day Cleansing Program

This program is designed to give the stomach a chance to cleanse itself and to give the other organs in the digestive chain time to remove waste buildup and to repair themselves. Consult Chapters 4 and 5 for general dietary considerations.

If you cannot follow this program exactly, it should not be undertaken, for adding regular amounts of food to Betonite may cause the food to jell in the alimentary tract and defeat the entire purpose of the cleansing. Do not take any supplements or vitamins.

Day One:

First thing upon awaking, take a coffee or chickory-root enema, according to instructions given in the chapter on detoxification.

Drink a half cup of Betonite (this is a diatomaceous earth in colloidal suspension, which acts to change the ionic balance in the intestinal tract, drawing toxins to it and eliminating them; its action is entirely mechanical, and it is not absorbed into the system). Most health food stores sell Betonite.

Juices should be freshly made, or may be purchased in bottles (not cans) and unpasteurized. Frozen juices are not acceptable.

FOOD

Breakfast. A six-ounce glass of fruit juice, such as apple or black cherry juice. Carrot juice or any green vegetable juice may be substituted if preferred.

10:00 A.M. Another six-ounce glass of fresh juice, preferably carrot.

Lunch. A fresh green salad, Romaine or Red Leaf lettuce (not head lettuce). Dressing may be of yogurt with some herbs such as chives, basil, or dill weed added for flavor.

3:00 P.M. A glass of fresh juice, followed by another half cup of Betonite with a glass of pure water.

Evening. Glass of fresh juice, as above.

Days Two and Three:

Same as day 1 above, except substitute for the luncheon salad a serving of lightly steamed shredded carrots (3 min.). Continue with enemas and Betonite.

Day Four:

Wake-up; take enema and Betonite.
Breakfast. Glass of fresh juice as on previous days.

10:00 A.M. Second glass of juice, preferably carrot.

Lunch. One cooked fresh green vegetable of choice or serving of lightly steamed shredded carrots.

3:00 P.M. Glass of fresh carrot juice, followed by half cup of Betonite and a glass of water.

Evening. Shredded carrots, lightly steamed, plus one cooked fresh green vegetable.

Day Five:

Wake-up; take enema and half cup of Betonite.

Resume regular diet as before cleansing program, but eat about one-third less than normal.

For many people this will seem too severe, but it is necessary to reduce radically the food intake and to supply cleansing fresh juices (carrot juice is a fine blood cleanser and purifier). There may well be such signs as a headache, perhaps even slight nausea, but it is only the body's own inner system working to cleanse itself. The chickory-root or coffee enemas are vital to keep the process of natural elimination going and to relieve the stress that will fall upon the main organs of elimination— the kidneys, spleen, and gall bladder.

Any attempt to rebuild the system completely by means of judicious diet should be supervised by a competent physician, preferably a naturopath or one who is familiar with natural kinds of therapy.

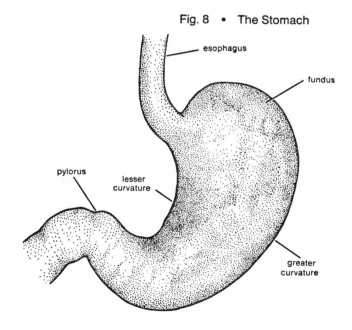

Fig. 8 • The Stomach

9.1 Bad Temperament of the Stomach

In a person with hot temperament, the softness of low-calorie foods causes the stomach to become foul. Hard food and food of high caloric value is the answer. Sometimes there is thirst caused by salty phlegm. This can be relieved by drinking warm water; cold water will not quench the thirst. However, if the cause is bile or excess internal heat, cold water will suffice.

9.2 Stomachache

If the cause of pain is gas, there is much belching and hiccups and the stomach is distended from the gas. When partially digested food reaches to the bottom of the stomach, pain is felt in the area of the spleen. Remedy: Apply a hot pack to the stomach and drink peppermint tea, with a few drops of rose oil added. Chewing pennyroyal is useful to cause belching and expel gas. If the gas is quite dense, use the phlegm purgative. An immediate effect is gained by applying cupping to the stomach. Honey and vinegar or anise-seed tea may also be used to relieve the pain of gaseousness.

Another cause of stomachache is prevalence of dense gas in the empty bowel. Another cause is that bile has poured into the stomach from the liver because the stomach has been empty for a long time. Another cause is that impure bile spills onto the cardia of the spleen. In the case of gas, use a purgative. For bile, adjust the bile humour and use a purgative, followed by cupping on the brachial artery of the right arm.

A ready-made formula for stomach distress and general cleansing of the stomach, which I have used and found to be the most effective of many, is available from Nature's Herb Company, 281 Ellis Street, San Francisco, California 94102. It is sold as Herbal Tea No. 285 and contains buckbean leaves, gentian root, wormwood herb, yarrow leaves, eriodictyon, licorice root, and cassia bark.

9.3 Weakness of Digestion

The sign of bad digestion is that the food comes out in the stools in an almost unchanged condition, or sometimes by vomiting or diarrhea. The food does not remain in the stomach more than a few hours. Ground fennel seed, with ginger, mixed in honey is the specific remedy for all cases of poor digestion.

9.4 Cholera

This disease causes corrupted substances to come to the stomach from various parts of the body and be emitted by vomiting or diarrhea. If the cholera is very severe, there is no vomiting, and all the substance is eliminated by diarrhea. The accompanying signs of fainting, lowered pulse, and occasional convulsions are not as dangerous as they seem. They can be reversed easily, especially in children. If cholera becomes chronic, it is dangerous, and is the leading cause of death among infants in underdeveloped nations. The remedy is to remove the corrupted substance completely. While it may seem illogical, one should try to increase the diarrhea or vomiting, as the body realizes that there is a toxic substance and is trying to eliminate it by the quickest route possible. Use laxatives and provoke vomiting by giving tincture of lobelia in teaspoon doses. If the person feels faint, give lemons to chew on. Restrict the diet to simple foods, ensure ample rest, keeping the patient in bed, because nothing works better than rest and fasting. Uncomplicated cholera is self-limiting, with recovery evident by the third to sixth day. Vaccines are available for cholera protection.

9.5 Deficient and Invalid Appetite

There are many causes. First, it can be bad temperament, whether excessively hot or cold, which affects the cardia. Second is the collection of phlegm in the stomach. Third is the body being filled with raw phlegm, which interferes with the normal appetitive signals of the body to the stomach. Fourth is density of skin pores and roughness of skin, which stop absorption. Fifth is that the liver is weak and obstruction occurs, either in the liver itself or in the mesentery. Sixth is that obstruction occurs in the valve between the spleen and the cardia. Seventh is that the nerve sensors in the cardia are impaired. (NOTE:

When the parts of the body need food, they "ask" the veins. The veins carry this message to the liver, which conveys this request to the mesentery, which alerts the stomach via a very sensitive nerve network in the cardia. At this time, bile is secreted from the spleen into the stomach, causing what we call hunger. If any part of this process is blocked, delayed, or altered, the sense of hunger is corrupted or fails.)

The remedies are as follows: *foul substances in the stomach*: purge; for *density of pores*: open by bathing and loofa scrubbing; for *liver weakness*: reinforce liver (see section 10.2, on the liver); for *obstruction of spleen*: purge spleen (see 11.4); and for *nerve failure in cardia*: reinforce the brain (see 2.2).

Sometimes anemia or quitting an addiction can slacken hunger. If there is deficient appetite over an extended period—a month or longer—the stomach is the seat of the anemia. Cure it by using foods and herbs that increase appetite, such as lemon juice, green spearmint, vinegar, onion, salty fish, sour pomegranate, and juice of pennyroyal.

9.6 Corrupted Appetite

Corrupted or inordinate appetite includes the desire for such things as mud or the tendency of the pregnant woman to crave a peculiar food, such as pickles. I once saw a woman who desired to eat cotton and paper. Ultimately, the cause is accumulation of corrupted phlegm in the stomach. Use a purgative, except in the case of pregnant women, who should take nothing, as these cravings will pass after three months without treatment.

9.7 Excessive Appetite

The person cannot satisfy his hunger, and wants to eat "like a dog." If the cause is a cold-natured temperament, the signs are insufficient thirst and intense gas. The remedy is to warm up the cardia by eating fresh hot bread and rubbing nutmeg and valerian on the stomach. If there is phlegm in the stomach, purge the stomach. If the cause is bile spilling on the cardia from the spleen, the signs are great hunger along with burning sensation on the cardia. The burning will not go away unless food is eaten. Purge the black bile humour and apply cupping over the spleen. If the cause is phlegm coming down from the brain into the stomach, the sign is that the food turns sour in the stomach, followed by much belching. Purge the brain.

9.8 Loss of Appetite

The person wants no food, not even one mouthful, in spite of the fact that the body needs nourishment. The signs are emaciation and loss of vitality. When this ailment lingers, it causes fainting. For fainting, consult the proper section. If the person is very weak, enemas are not advised. Instead, reinforce the stomach (see 9.2, 9.3).

9.9 Impatient Hunger

The person acts as though he won't be able to refrain from eating and seems always to be hunting for something to eat. Reinforce the cardia by feeding apple juice and subacid pomegranate juice (not too sour).

9.10 Severe Thirst

There are two kinds: true thirst and false thirst. True thirst is that which is experienced to offset heat. Signs of the effect of heat and dryness are apparent, and the person benefits from cold water. This is normal desire. False thirst occurs when salty phlegm and burning canker collect in the stomach and the temperament needs water to wash these away. The signs are that the body is not relieved by cold water, and the taste in the mouth is changed. In this case, breathing cold air and inhaling cold-natured substances are useful. If there are signs that the person has cold-natured substances in the stomach, he should vomit after drinking warm water with honey and vinegar. Afterward, feed anise water, chicken, and pea water. Eating garlic and honey is also effective.

In the case of salty phlegm caused by excess internal heat,

allow only anise water or a little sweet almond oil. If the cause is swelling of the liver or fever, consult the sections on those problems.

9.11 Swelling of the Stomach

If the cause is cold-natured substances in the stomach, the person is slightly feverish. If it is from hot-natured substances, there is high fever and pain. Remedy: In hot nature, cup the stomach but do not give strong laxatives, and induce vomiting. If there is constipation, give purging cassia, tamarind, and red clover tea. An external pomade made of sandalwood and common scallions is recommended. After three days of this, change the pomade to one composed of barley flower, marshmallow, and rose water.

For cold-natured corruption, make the pomade of sweet flag root and cooked hyssop. If the cause is black bile humour, give willow oil mixed with purging cassia decoction for three days.

9.12 Corruption of Stomach Juices into Rheum

If the cause is swelling of the liver, the remedy calls for ripening the rheum with a pomade made of bitter almond, willow oil, and mastic and have the person drink plenty of warm water to assist ripening. If the rheum ripens by itself, it is fine. After three days of ripening, clean it out with goat's milk and honey water. After cleaning, drink tea of pomegranate blossoms and dragon's-blood.

9.13 Ulcers and Boils of the Stomach

The sign is severe pain immediately after eating sour or hot foods. The location of the pain reveals whether the ulcer is in the cardia or lower part of the stomach. Apply the remedies found in 9.11 according to the signs, or give buttermilk with a little magnesia, red clover blossoms, and sour grape seeds.

In the case of boils, use the remedy for swelling of the

stomach, but never forget to use an enema. For a laxative, use cassia with syrup of chickory. If the stomach seems loose, give magnesia with barley bran.

9.14 Stomach Gas

The cause is bad cold temperament or corruption of the food in the stomach, or collection of phlegm in the stomach. See 9.1 and 9.3 for weak digestion and bad temperament. Fennel seed boiled in rose water is very useful.

9.15 Belching, Yawning, and Gasping

These are caused by excess gas. Remedy: Use a purgative and correct digestion. Relief of gas can be had from musk oil, mastic with honey, or ground anise in rose water.

9.16 Vomiting and Nausea

What is expelled forcibly via the mouth is called vomiting. If you have the desire to vomit and can't, it is called nausea. Use the purgative for the phlegm humour. To cause vomiting, use a teaspoon of tincture of lobelia every ten minutes until the effect is secured; or, for a less violent emetic, drink lukewarm water ($\frac{3}{4}$ glass) with honey (1 tablespoon) and vinegar (5 tablespoons).

To stop vomiting caused by biliousness, give mixture of amber, dates, tamarind, purslane, magnesia, and barley bran, each one dram.

To stop vomiting from phlegm imbalance and to reinforce the stomach take aloe wood, ground clove, pennyroyal, mastic, each one dram, and add to ten drams of rose preserve. Pound and sift together, and give one dram of the compound with ten drams of rose water.

A pomade recommended for vomiting caused by black bile humour imbalance is: watercress, moss, myrtle leaves, and white clover, in equal parts, plus a little honey for texture, placed on the spleen.

Cupping close to the navel and between the shoulders and vigorous massage also have a good effect to stop vomiting.

9.17 Vomiting Blood

There are two sources: one is that a vein from the gullet or stomach is pierced or broken. It is known by a recent injury to the gullet or stomach. If there is pain between the shoulders, it is a sign that there is an ulcer in the gullet or stomach. Binding the arms and cupping the legs are recommended, as is eating large, seeded raisins to help congest the vein openings.

The other source of vomited blood is due to an internal injury or other calamity to the liver, spleen, or head, and blood is poured into the stomach and thrown off. Emergency medical aid must be sought as soon as possible.

If there is a crushing chest injury and emergency medical aid is not available, this remedy is given: acacia, ammonia salt, aloe vera juice, and myrrh (in equal parts) mixed with myrtle water; place over the affected organ.

9.18 Clotting of Blood

When blood spills into the stomach from an internal source and is not expelled due to lack of internal heat, it forms a clot. The signs that this has happened are that cold sweat and fainting appear and the person trembles. Remedy: Boil half an ounce each of common dill weed and pennyroyal, along with a half ounce of honey and the same amount of vinegar, and drink hot.

9.19 Milk in the Stomach

It often happens that milk is coagulated in a nursing baby's stomach due to the illness of the mother. Give the baby a few ounces of pennyroyal tea to open the coagulated milk. Adjust the mother's food during illness and give relaxing teas, such as peppermint, to both mother and baby. During the mother's illness, never feed the baby fully.

9.20 Hiccups

Mild hiccups after eating will pass without drastic treatment. If they persist for several hours, the cause must be determined and treated accordingly. If the cause is overeating, it happens immediately after the meal; remove the food with an emetic and correct the digestion.

If the vomiting continues after the food is expelled, take a decoction of pennyroyal.

If the cause is gas, which is common with babies, the hiccups occur after eating gas-producing foods. The remedy for gas is given in 9.14.

Hiccups can also be caused by excess of phlegm. If this is the case, induce vomiting with honey and vinegar or lobelia, and adjust the digestion with fresh fruit juices and milk. Drinking warm water and one tablespoon of plain almond oil or butter with meals will have the same effect.

Another cause of hiccups is that moisture of phlegm has adhered to the surface of the stomach lining. The signs of this are watery mouth, sour belching, and incomplete digestion. The remedy is to use an enema.

If the cause of hiccups is bad cold nature of temperament, the signs are sleepiness, cold hands, and low pulse and are corrected by eating hot-natured foods.

If the cause is due to swelling of the liver or stomach, consult 9.11 and 10.7.

Making a person sneeze is quite effective in relieving hiccups. Sniff some black pepper. Other remedies include drinking a tea of pennyroyal with juice of sour pomegranate and lots of icy-cold water. Cooked cinnamon and mastic are also mentioned as effective, as is holding the breath for as long as possible.

9.21   Vomiting after Food Is Digested

The cause of this is usually that there are lesions in the intestine—when the intestine is unable to assimilate food, it must be gotten rid of (ejected) by vomiting. The remedy is given in 13.2.

9.22   Upset Stomach

The person feels a kind of "fearful churning" of the stomach, similar to the sensation when confronting a dangerous situation, right after eating. Use a phlegm purgative and drink peppermint tea.

9.23 Convulsion of the Stomach

There is a throbbing movement in the cardia. Remedy: Use a
phlegm humour purgative. The cause may also be worms,
which must be removed. Presence of parasites can be detected
by iridology.

9.24 Heartache

Severe pain is felt in the cardia. The hands become cold and
clammy and the person may faint. Remedy: Consult section on
stomachache.

9.25 Heartburn, or Stomach Burn

If the cause of the burning sensation is from eating unleavened
bread or green fruit or imprisonment of raw moisture in the
stomach, eating moist foods will correct it. Remedy: Reinforce
the digestion (see 9.2).
   The cause may also be from black bile humour imbalance.
If so, cup on the right or left arm, then give dates, jams, and
honey. Drink fennel tea with a quarter-teaspoon of ground
ginger added.

9.26 Slackness of the Stomach

There are two kinds: one is in the nature of the stomach. Its
signs are poor digestion and projection of the chest. The other
type of slackness relates to the parts that connect to the stomach.
Apply what was given in the sections on slackness (2.19) and
paralysis (2.18) and feed soft foods. Allow the person to inhale
sweet flowers and use astringent herbs.

9.27 Slackness of the Stomach Tissues

This is a degeneration of tissue that involves all parts of the
stomach, and is the worst stomach affliction. The signs are false
or incomplete digestion, despite eating very soft foods, and
constipation. Rub the stomach with amber oil and mastic. Feed
only fowl. It will take a long time and wise guidance from a
physician to relieve this affliction.

9.28 Hardness of the Stomach

This hard swelling occurs mostly in the area of the cardia and can be felt, so no other signs are necessary. If the swelling is severe enough, it can even be seen. The cause is usually imbalance of the hot temperament. Apply cupping on the veins of the arms and make a salve of white wax, bitter almond, balsam, chicken fat, and everything that will absorb phlegm. Especially recommended is iodine, available in pure kelp and sea food or as organic iodine from a physician.

It sometimes occurs that due to hardness of the spleen, coarseness is felt in parts of the stomach. See also 11.1.

9.29 Hardness of the Stomach Muscles

Such hardness happens in the lengthwise striations of the muscle fibers. The remedy is the same as for bad, hot intemperament of the stomach (9.1).

9.30 Stomach Corruption

This can be caused from bad temperament and is treated in 9.1. The cause can also be an ulcer or boil, discussed in 9.13. Another cause is called brain diarrhea and is signaled by continuous diarrhea. The person usually falls asleep for a twelve- or fourteen-hour period, and the signs do not reappear for a long time. The true remedy is given in the chapter on the head and brain.

In this latter case, never try to stop the diarrhea. The remedy is in correcting the diet and improving digestion. If the cause is weakness of the liver, the sign is gradually increasing weakness. Remedy: Reinforce the liver and stomach, and take some mastic with a diet plentiful in fresh green vegetables.

9.31 Smallness of the Stomach

The stomach can naturally become smaller due to decreased intake of food over a period of time. If this is the case, ingesting large amounts of food at one sitting can be harmful, even if the food is soft, for the stomach is not accustomed to the quantity. The stomach may also be shriveled because of convulsion or swelling, as discussed in 9.11 and 9.23.

9.32 Stomach Flu

The sign of the heat of flu is the softness of the feces. The sign of flu from cold intemperament is thickness of the matter coming out of the nose. The remedy is to adjust the temperament and endure the symptoms. Eat soft foods, keep the body warm and the head covered. Avoid lying flat on the back, eating sour things, milk, or meat.

The Liver

General Considerations

The liver is a compound tubular gland located in the upper right part of the abdominal cavity immediately below the diaphragm. It is the largest gland of the body, weighing about 1500 grams.

The main functions of the liver are secretion of bile, formation of blood, metabolic functions, detoxification, and a thermal function. Two of these functions—regulation of blood volume and production of heat—make this the most important organ from the view of natural medicine. (While the liver produces bile, this substance is stored in the gall bladder.) Some researchers believe that the liver can accomplish reoxidations and metabolic regenerations.

The functions of the liver are so vitally important for the body that they can be compared with the activity of chlorophyll in plants. Indeed, the liver is so crucial biologically that it can be called the balance of the wheel of life. Dr. Max Gerson, one of the pioneers of nontoxic cancer therapy, concluded that the recovery possibility in cancer depends directly on the degree of damage to liver function. The liver can remain damaged for a long time because the deterioration of the liver cannot be detected before its great functional reserves have been consumed. The liver has great capacity to regenerate. Therefore, a partial destruction may be restored if deterioration is not extensive and rapid.

The great difficulty is to determine when pathological destruction of the liver actually begins. For this purpose, the science of iridology is useful in evaluating the degree of liver degeneration.

In view of the unanimous agreement among all medical systems new and old on the supreme place the liver holds in human health, it is easy to see why all concern should be exercised to avoid any activities or substances that interfere with correct liver function.

One of the main conditions that affects the liver is cirrhosis, as it is called by Western medicine. It is well known that excessive consumption of alcohol in any form may lead to cirrhosis; it is also well worth considering the potential benefits to health and longevity of restriction of consumption of alcoholic beverages. Excessive drinking (which can be the two or three martinis of the "social" drinker) often carries other patterns of living with it, such as lack of exercise, anxiety from high-stress vocations, large consumption of meat and fats, and high coronary-disease risks, among others.

10.1 Bad Temperament of the Liver

All the *hakims* I consulted were in agreement that chickory is the best remedy for bad temperament of the liver. Adding

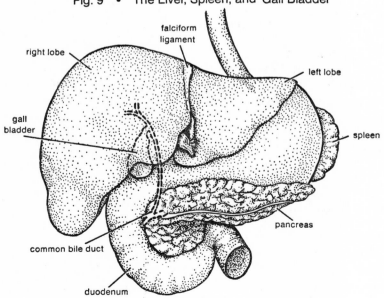

Fig. 9 • The Liver, Spleen, and Gall Bladder

falciform ligament

right lobe

left lobe

gall bladder

spleen

common bile duct

pancreas

duodenum

purgative cassia is also recommended if the cause is any kind of substance obstructing the liver. When there is constipation, give laxatives and cold-natured substances such as pomegranate juice and sandalwood syrup. To these can be added honey and vinegar, barberry water, and cold buttermilk. If the stomach is soft and queasy, drink astringent teas such as yellow dock or bayberry and magnesia with quince or apple conserve.

If imbalance of the blood humour is the cause of liver intemperament and there is no obstruction of the liver, cup the veins on the arms. If the cause is biliousness, putting cold-natured compresses on the liver will reduce the overheating. Cucumber works well.

If the person has diarrhea, give purslane seeds, sweet basil seeds, and gum Arabic, one teaspoon of each. Fry these together for ten minutes in a little oil, soak in rose water, and take a teaspoon several times a day.

To purge the black bile humour affecting the liver, moistening medicines are required; apply a salve of cooked rose leaves and give a tea made from equal parts of rose hips, cowslip, mint, and anise. Be careful not to use this preparation for more than two days, for too much moisture can lead to dropsy.

10.2   Weakness of the Liver

While many things can weaken the liver, the signs are the foul odor of the urine as it is emitted and its color, which is like the water one would have from washing fresh meat. The appetite is lessened, and there may be general weakness. The person may complain of pain on the right side just below the last rib, especially after eating. The face color may be of a greenish tint, or sometimes yellowish. Give coffee or chickory-root enemas, and apply the remedy from 10.1 according to the signs.

10.3   Obstruction of the Liver

The tissues of the liver, or the blood vessels supplying the liver, are obstructed with phlegm. The signs of this are a lessened production of blood in the body, yellow face, diarrhea, and a feeling of heaviness in the liver. If the obstruction is in the convex portion of the liver, more heaviness is felt, and reduced amounts of thin urine are excreted. If the obstruction is in the concave part, much thick, moist feces are passed. The difference between obstruction and swelling of the liver is that in the case of swelling there is fever and pain. In obstruction, there is seldom pain and more heaviness is felt.

Remedy: First, coffee or chickory-root enemas. Also, if the obstruction is in the convex part of the liver, give diuretics; if in the concave portion, use laxatives. Watch the diet carefully, and add fresh liver juice. If the obstruction is caused by eating astringent foods, it may be removed by eating such things as milk, sugar, almond oil, and pomegranate.

Obstruction may also be caused by narrowness of the blood vessels of the liver; this is usually apparent from childhood. The remedy is to drink diuretics and to avoid eating hot and energetic foods.

10.4 Gas of the Liver

The first sign is that pain is felt under the right rib. No heaviness is felt in the liver, and there is no fever. After digestion of food, the gas increases. Eat millet, take warm baths at noon, and keep warm packs over the place where pain is felt. Give laxatives and diuretics, and follow the remedy for gas in the stomach (see 9.1, 9.3, and 9.14).

10.5 Liver Ache

The causes are bad temperament, gas, or swelling, discussed above.

10.6 Liver Pain after Drinking Cold Water

For some reason, this most often occurs before noon, and after getting out of a warm bath. The remedy is to soak half an ounce of purslane in warm water, and apply as a poultice to the liver. A pomade of hyacinth and mastic is also recommended. This pain soon goes away, but has to be treated if it recurs, as it can lead to dropsy.

10.7 Swelling of the Liver

If the cause is improper blood or bile humour, the signs are fever, thirst, heaviness of stomach, pain in area of the liver, vomiting, fainting, coldness in extremities, asthma, and retention of urine (or some combination of these signs). The remedy in cases of blood humour imbalance is to apply cupping on the right arm, followed by chickory water and pomegranate juice mixed with a little vinegar and honey. If there is any constipation, give laxatives, and always remember chickory enemas.

If the cause is inharmony of the bile humour, apply the same remedy as for blood humour, but follow with a pomade made of barley flour, sandalwood, rose water, chickory, and vinegar (in equal parts).

If the cause is phlegm humour inharmony, the signs are extreme heavy feeling, a salty taste of phlegm in the mouth, and a very slight pain in the liver, but no fever. Laxatives are advised.

A feeling of hardness is a sign that black bile humour is affected and must be adjusted. After the canker has been softened, milk with a little sugar can be given to good effect if there is no high temperature.

If the liver is swelling due to a blow to the body or a fall, apply this pomade: grind and sift three drams of peas with the skins removed (soaking for fifteen minutes in water will assist easy removal) and two drams of beeswax. Mix these with oil of violet for consistency.

10.8 Large, Round Swelling of Liver

Apply what was recommended for bad temperament (10.1) and follow with the remedy for swelling of the stomach (9.11). If the swelling is inclined downward toward the intestines, give a light purgative. If it is inclined toward the kidneys, give a diuretic. If the swelling tends toward the interior of the body, it is a warning sign of dropsy.

If the cause of swelling is relieved by these measures, the signs will go away, even though no rheum of phlegm passes in the urine or feces. It is difficult to determine whether the corrupted substance may have been dumped into the interior of the body.

10.9 Boils on Surface of Liver

The sign of boils is the appearance of red marks on the skin over the area of the liver, which proves there is hot, burning intemperament of the liver. The remedy is the same as prescribed for bad intemperament of the liver (10.1).

10.10 Palpitation of the Liver

The liver palpitates in convulsive movements, and there is a feeling as if someone were blowing on the liver. This condition goes away soon. Its cause is a slight obstruction of the liver, which can often relieve itself. Apply reflex massage of the feet.

10.11 Liver Stones

The sign of stones forming in the liver is that after eating there is vomiting and pain is felt in the liver. Swelling can be felt by touch, and sometimes can be seen. There is a peculiar "sandy" quality to the blood, if it is drawn and examined. Consult the remedy in 14.9 for kidney stones.

10.12 Shrinking of Liver

The causes and signs are the same as for smallness of the stomach. Purge the liver with coffee enemas, laxatives, and diuretics.

10.13 Diarrhea of the Liver

There are five forms of this ailment: (1) Caused by rupture during swelling of the liver. Consult the remedy in 9.11 on swollen stomach. (2) Urine of a watery pink color, which is caused by chronic degeneration of the liver. The remedy for this form is the same as for liver weakness (10.2). (3) Caused by blood. This is called *zusentar* in Persian, a derivative from the Greek word that means stomach ulcer. Its cause is an excess fullness of blood manufactured by the liver, without any internal broken blood vessels. (If the cause is from an internal injury or falling down or similar things, blood comes out continuously from the rectum. Any case of internal bleeding needs the immediate attention of a physician. It is not good to stop the flow of blood, as it may back up and inflate the kidneys.) Use enemas to assist elimination if no medical help is available. It is felt advisable to constipate the system to stem excessive flow of blood; amber, syrup of purslane, and mother's milk are recommended, a teaspoon of each. (4) Caused by biliousness. The sign of this condition is the red pocklike marks over the liver area indicating excessive heating of the liver, and thus overproduction of bile. Apply the remedy for bad temperament of the liver (10.1). (5) Serum. This is caused by burning of blood and phlegm in the liver. Removing bile with a laxative is necessary. Afterward, apply a pomade made of sandalwood and rose water on the heart and liver.

10.14   Dropsy

There are three kinds: (1) the bowel is projected because there are impacted substances in it; (2) the bowel and other parts of the body are distended due to water accumulating in the layers of the bowel (it can also be due to gas distention, in which case the bowel sounds like a drum when you tap on it); and (3) heat of the liver. In the latter case, apply the remedy found in 10.1.

For dropsy, use of laxatives and diuretics is recommended, along with methods to open up external elimination such as using steam baths, dry heat, and hot pomades. Avoid anything of a hot nature in foods, and also avoid an extreme of coldness. Drink only pure water to which anise or chickory has been added. These should be sipped plentifully during the day and at each meal. Reduce the amount of food eaten to one-sixth the amount normally eaten. The most useful single food is pomegranate; eat as much as you like. Meat-eaters should concentrate on white meat of chicken, lamb, and green vegetables such as peas. Cereals and grains should be avoided as much as possible. If they are demanded, give only rice. In dropsy types 1 and 2, use coffee enemas and keep up with diuretics, changing the herbs from time to time since the body will gradually become immune to its efforts. If you consume herbs in capsules, grind them very fine first so that they will take immediate effect.

To induce perspiration, lie in a bath or other suitable place. Rub salt mixed with a little oil over the body. Then cover with soft sand. If the sand is cold, add more, as much as can be tolerated, as this takes the swelling away. Usually only a part of the body is treated in this way (rather than the whole body). If sand is not available, sitting with the back exposed to the sun for fifteen to thirty minutes, or bathing in warm fresh springs or mineral baths will have the same effect. The best treatment is bathing in the sea. If there is no sea water, put sun-evaporated sea salt in distilled water for three or four days and expose to the sun. This will make an acceptable substitute for sea water. Some health food stores sell a product called Nigari, which has the therapeutic properties of sea water.

For the second kind of dropsy mentioned, distension due to accumulated water, boil 100 parts of water with one part of very old grape vinegar. Boil until reduced to one-third, cool, and drink. If there is coughing, do not give sour things. A pomade is also recommended for this form of dropsy, as follows: turbinado sugar, lily of the valley root, each 3 drams; beet seeds, 7 drams; barley flower, 60 drams. Grind and mix with anise water or chickory water and apply to belly.

When dropsy is chronic, as known by the "drum" sound on tapping, the hardness of the liver will increase, even though the person feels better. There is no problem except the swelling of the belly. This is the time to use softening pomades. When the hardness is softened, make this mixture and apply to the belly to absorb the substance: Pound together feverfew herb, white clover, seeds of wild rue, castoreum, white rose (each one-sixth ounce), and mix with rue water to make a pomade.

The Spleen and Gall Bladder

11.1 Jaundice

The main disease of the spleen is jaundice. It occurs in two main forms, characterized by either yellow skin (imbalance of the yellow bile humour) or blackened skin (black bile humour). The black form originates in the spleen itself, while the yellow type is generally caused by malfunction of the liver and gall bladder. Yellow jaundice will be discussed first.

11.2 Yellow Jaundice

1. The severe form of yellow jaundice occurs *as a complication of other illness*. The nature of the body is to expel toxic matters, so if the skin is yellow, it is a good sign that there is no failure of organ function. Bathe in warm water, drink honey and vinegar or chickory syrup, and the color will go away by itself.

2. Another form of yellow jaundice is caused by *bad temperament of the liver*. This must be treated according to 10.1.

3. *Hot temperament of the gall bladder* also causes the sign of yellowing skin. The sign that this is the problem is that it comes on suddenly, and the urine is white in color, changing a few days later to dark yellow and finally to a dark, almost brown color. There is no sign of bad temperament of the liver or obstruction. The person has a good appetite. Give honey and vinegar with chickory syrup.

4. Yellow jaundice caused by *swelling of the gall bladder* is

evidenced by fever, vomiting, roughness of the tongue, and nausea. Apply the remedy given in 10.7.

5. Yellow skin is also a sign of *extreme high temperature* of the whole body. The signs are feeling the heat of the skin by touch and constipation of the bowels. If the cause is from simple excess heat, give cold foods and herbs; if it is from a corrupt substance in the body, use purgatives and general adjustment of the diet.

6. Another cause of yellowing is *obstruction of the pores,* from traveling without protection for long periods of time under a hot sun and from dust covering the skin. Open the pores by washing with cooked violet flowers, white clover, chrysanthemums, marshmallow, and bran (in equal parts).

7. Yellow jaundice is also caused by a *poisonous insect sting or from eating poisonous drugs or foods.* The skin is activated as an organ of elimination in such an emergency. First, remove the effect. Then see sections on insect bites and poisoning (21.27). Seek emergency first aid for any accidental poisoning or serious insect or animal bite.

8. *Weakness of gall bladder* can cause yellow jaundice. The gall bladder becomes weak and cannot absorb bile from the liver, finally resulting in jaundice. The signs are vomiting, constipation, and yellow feces. See 10.2 for remedy.

9. *Obstruction of the vessel connection between the gall bladder and the liver* also causes jaundice. The feces gradually lighten in color until they are almost white. See next paragraph and the remedy given in 10.2.

10. *Obstruction between the gall bladder and intestine* will also cause the feces to become white suddenly, along with a great sense of constipation. The remedy is an enema to remove the obstruction. In both cases of obstruction dissolve a teaspoon of powdered purging cassia in water of beets, mix with six or eight ground apricot kernels (sweet, not bitter ones), and take a tablespoon twice a day.

11. *Fleshy growth over organ valves.* Additional tissue sometimes grows over an outlet for no known reason. Sometimes it is present from birth, congenital. There is no natural cure; sometimes the impairment can be corrected by surgery.

12. Jaundice is also caused by a kind of *phlegm colic,* due to

very watery phlegm blocking the mouth of the vein going to the stomach. This is the place that bile enters the stomach. The remedy is to remove the colic.

If you want to remove the yellowness from the eyes during jaundice, inhale some stale vinegar in a warm bath and put a few drops of rose water, vinegar, and sour pomegranate juice in the eyes.

11.3 Black Jaundice

1. The bad temperament of the *spleen causes lymph fluid to be thrown off.* This is very severe and spleen diseases follow. The remedy is to assist nature in its elimination, as was mentioned in 10.13(4). Also massage with oil of feverfew herb.

2. *Obstruction of outlet between spleen and cardia;* or

3. *Obstruction of outlet between the liver and spleen* are both recognized by these signs: the jaundice appears slowly, the liver is heavy, and the appetite gradually diminishes. Open the obstruction by taking laxatives.

4. *Burning of blood* due to excess heat in liver. Consult 10.1.

5. *Weakness of the spleen* is seen in the signs of loss of appetite and the whites of the eyes becoming swollen. The signs of weakness of self-regulating faculty of the spleen are excretion of black bile by vomiting and diarrhea.

6. Caused by bad and *excessive cold temperament of the liver.* The remedy is given in 10.1.

If jaundice is both yellow and black, apply cupping on the veins of both arms every three days. Soften the stomach by drinking teas for yellow or black bile. Correct the temperament of the liver and the spleen. Foods recommended to strengthen the spleen are lemon juice, citrus, green pepper, and buckwheat.

11.4 Bad Temperament of the Spleen

The signs are burning of the spleen and redness or blackness of urine and feces if the cause is heat. If the cause is cold, there is stomach grumbling and lack of hunger. If there is dryness, the spleen is hard, the blood is thick, and the body generally weak. If due to moisture imbalance in the spleen, the signs are heaviness in the area of the spleen, and the body color is ashen.

If the cause is heat, this remedy is useful: nightshade, water of willow leaves, and water of wormwood with honey and vinegar (half a teaspoon each). For softening the hardness of the spleen, give cooked dates and purging cassia tea. Give cold foods as well.

In case of cold intemperament of the spleen, give celery water with honey and vinegar, or mix two parts grape juice with one part water and reduce to half by boiling; add a teaspoon of rose water and give in the mornings.

For dryness, violet syrup is recommended.

If the cause is corrupt substances in the spleen, laxatives are advised.

For moisture imbalance, make pills from red clover blossoms, hyacinth, and barberry herbs and take two several times a day.

11.5 Swelling of the Spleen

If the cause is heat, there is fever. If the cause is phlegm, there is convulsion of the spleen. In black bile or canker, the spleen is hard.

Remedies: For heat, make a pomade of barley flour and water of valerian.

For phlegm, make a pomade of rose oil and wood ash (or activated charcoal), two parts each:

a. mix with one part vinegar;
b. or, mix pennyroyal and wild rue with a little vinegar;
c. or, boil an ounce of bran in vinegar, add a few drops of ammonia

and make a pomade of it.

The *hakims* also recommend eating only from wooden bowls for forty days. For those suffering from a hardened spleen, it is recommended to apply cupping on the veins of the right arm.

11.6 Detoxifying the Spleen

Swelling of the spleen usually goes away by itself or becomes hard; it rarely ripens and becomes rheum. If it does become rheum, the rheum enters the stomach and is thrown off by vomiting or diarrhea. The remedy is given in 10.8. Adjust the temperament by giving diuretics.

If hardness remains after detoxifying, use the pomade in 11.5 for swelling of canker, and generally avoid using astringents. When hard swelling becomes chronic, it requires surgery.

11.7   Weakness of the Spleen

If the weakness is due to absorption of spleen fluids, there is no appetite. If it is from lack of self-control, there is diarrhea and vomiting. If it is from bad digestion, there is good appetite and diarrhea. To reinforce the spleen, make this pomade and apply to the spleen: hyacinth, caraway, tamarisk, red clover blossoms (in equal parts); grind and mix with wild rue water and vinegar and apply.

11.8   Obstructions of the Spleen

This is caused by weakness of the digestion. Remedy: Reinforce the spleen. Make a fomentation of wheat bran and salt, and add to a pomade made of turbinado sugar, pennyroyal, wild rue (in equal parts); add honey and vinegar for consistency. Apply cupping over the spleen.

11.9   Spleen Stones

The sign is a sandy granulation coming out with the urine and prickling sensation of the spleen. Eat lots of figs and apply the measures given in section 14.9.

The Anus

12.1 About Hemorrhoids

These are extra skin flaps filled with swollen blood vessels, appearing along the edges of the anus. One kind is called tree-like because it has many roots. Another kind is called date stone, and causes corruption of the blood humour. Sometimes hemorrhoids are caused by an imbalance of the bile humour. Generally burning and pain are the signs of biliousness and blood causes; pain and a prickling itch are the signs of thickened blood humour. Apply cupping on the inside of the buttocks, soften the stomach, and correct the blood humour. If there is bleeding, rub some amber oil on the anus.

If hemorrhoids are painful but there is no bleeding, make a fomentation of marshmallow and common dill, apply for half an hour at a time, and rub the anus area with peach oil. Then make a suppository of onion decoction, and use it also for enemas, to purify and cleanse the area of toxins. Hemorrhoids can usually be soothed simply by applying a flower oil. Surgical removal is sometimes recommended, but the hemorrhoids do grow back in some cases.

12.2 Flatulency

Flatulency means a thick gaseousness produced in the intestines, and it is painful. The gas sometimes goes down and is emitted as farting; other times it recedes back into the bowels or is trapped for a time in bowel pockets. There may be slight bleeding, diarrhea, and also grumbling of the lower bowels.

Use the black bile purgative, and take gas-relieving remedies (see 13.6). Massage, taking warm baths, and cupping the veins of the arm is recommended.

12.3 Anus Ulcer

This has its beginning as a lesion on the interior surface, toward the intestines. There is bile being secreted consistently. First press the ulcer to take out the bile, then use a suppository (soak it in gum Arabic decoction first). If the ulcer is in the intestine proper and gas and feces are emitted via the ulcer, it is a dangerous condition that needs expert medical attention.

12.4 Swelling of the Anus

Caused by intemperament of heat, the anus is inflamed and painful. Apply cupping between the buttocks. Apply white of egg mixed with arnicated oil. If it is very painful, grind some marijuana seeds and add to the mixture. Vomiting is said to have great beneficial effect.

12.5 Cracks in the Anus

This pertains to cracks of the lips of the anus on the outer, exposed surface. Avoid drinking very cold water or sour things. Try to keep the bowels soft and moving easily. Give syrup of violet, almond oil, and decoction of quince seeds and plenty of laxative foods.

12.6 Slackness of the Sphincter Muscle

The sign is the unintentional expulsion of gas. Remedy: Purge the bowels with enemas.

12.7 Protrusion of the Anus

If the cause is swelling, treat by cooking a quarter-ounce of marshmallow and the same amount of violet; mix in olive oil and apply to the anus while pushing the protruded part back into the rectum. If the cause is slackness of the sphincter, the sign is that the anus protrusion goes in and out quite easily. Rub arnicated oil on the anus and make a powder of pomegranate flower and apply to the anus.

12.8   Itching of the Anus

The cause may be small worms, which is treated by oxygen colonic irrigation by a physician. If the cause is phlegm, use a phlegm purgative and apply cupping on the coccyx. Rub the anus with an ounce of vinegar mixed with half an ounce of rose oil to relieve itching. Essential oil of wormwood is effective in ten-drop doses. Consumption of pumpkin seeds is also said to remove worms.

The Intestines

General Considerations

The small intestine has three digestive juices: pancreatic juice, intestinal juices, and bile. The fist two help complete digestion by the effect of various enzymes on the food. Bile, while not a digestive juice, serves an important function by emulsifying fats and aiding in excretion of waste products.

By the time food reaches the large intestine, the digestible materials have been acted upon by the enzymes and are nearing the stage of elimination as end products. The main functions of the large intestine, then, are absorption of water and elimination of waste products.

The consistency of semi-fluid chyme when it leaves the stomach through the illeocaecal valve remains about the same through the rest of digestion. Feces leaving the rectum are semi-solid, indicating that the large intestine absorbs a very considerable amount of water.

The fluid secreted by the intestines is thick and full of mucus. Foreign substances, including drugs, are eliminated by the intestines.

Large numbers of bacteria are usually consumed with the food eaten. Most of these are destroyed by the sterilizing and digestive action of the acids in the stomach, but some pass through unaffected and appear in the large intestines.

The principal changes brought about by bacteria in the intestines are fermentations. Carbohydrates are decomposed, with alcohol and acid products as a result. Proteins are also acted upon, giving rise to putrefactive products that include amines, volatile acids, and several gases (H_2S, H_2, CO_2, and CH_4). These are primarily responsible for the characteristic odor of feces.

Some of the amines are toxic, but usually have no effect upon the body, for even if absorbed into the body, they are rendered harmless by the detoxifying action of the liver. If intestinal putrefaction is excessive, if the mucus is hard and thick, or if the liver is weak and unable to perform its detoxifying action well, toxic products of digestion may enter the general circulation of the blood stream and produce toxic effects.

13.1 Food Passing Quickly through the Intestines

The cause may be boils in the *inner* surface of the intestines, the symptoms of which are heat in the abdomen, a feeling of pain when the food reaches the intestines, and emission of bile with the stools. The remedy is to adjust the yellow bile humour and use cold drinks and enemas for relief.

If the cause is boils on the *outer* surface of the intestines, itching is felt in the intestine and pain is felt in the area of the navel and the sides of the body. Food comes out undigested. Remedy: Apply a pomade of cold-natured herbs under the navel.

If the cause is moisture covering the inner surface of the intestine, moisture coming out with undigested food in the stools is the sign. Remedy: Vomiting with emetics, and coffee or chickory-root enemas.

The intestine can become befouled with accumulated toxins and cause bad temperament of the intestine. Signs of moisture appear (sweating, tears), but no moisture is excreted with the stools. Use coffee or chickory-root enemas, very light-acting herbs, and rub rose oil on the abdomen.

If the cause is phlegm, the passing of mucus is noticed, and the person may desire to eat fruits before his meals. Use coffee or chickory-root enemas and increase the intake of iodine by eating kelp, watercress, and lots of greens and dates. Eliminate sugars, fruits, and bread. This herbal medicine is useful: yellow date, 2 drams; myrtle, sumac, and parsley, 4 grams ground each. Pound and add honey water to make a syrup. Take one teaspoon with meals.

If weakness is felt in the intestine because of paralysis or slackness of the peristaltic action, consult the section on paralysis (2.20).

13.2 Diarrhea Caused by Bleeding in the Intestine

There are two forms: one is from internal scratches of the intestine; the other is that the nerves of the intestine are engorged with blood, and the ending of one or more of the nerves is raw and bleeding.

Intestinal scratches One of the causes of this is from eating refined salt and sugars. When these are processed, the extreme heat causes the molecular structure to change so that they cannot be completely liquified. The resultant crystals are like minute glass particles that scratch and damage the interior of the intestines. It can also be caused by bile irritation over a long period, and the sign is diarrhea. The treatment at the beginning of the signs is to drink plenty of grape juice (if you can make your own from green grapes, it is better). Pomegranate juice and sour, astringent things such as sauerkraut and strawberries are good. If there is constipation, plantain enemas are recommended.

If the cause is phlegm, diarrhea with phlegm occurs, along with flu and catarrh of the bowels. Use an emetic, and then make an infusion from fresh basil seeds, along with black dates fried in safflower oil, and take three pills formed from this mixture twice a day.

If the cause of intestinal scratches is black bile, the sign is continuous gripe, and appearance of hardened mucus mixed with blood in the feces. After adjusting the black bile humour, reinforce the spleen (see 11.4) and give laxatives.

If the cause is excess of dryness in the intestine, the sign is constipation. Give moistening foods like quince, and take syrup of violet with almond oil. Use enemas. When the intestine is clear of digested foods, give astringent medicine, but never give astringents before cleaning out the colon.

If the irritation of the intestine is due to taking too many laxatives, stop them and drink plenty of buttermilk.

The second cause of diarrhea is *irritation of the nerve endings in the intestines*. Its sign is slight emission of blood with diarrhea of the stools, but there are no signs of diarrhea of the liver and no hemorrhoids. There is usually no pain. It is opposite to the signs for the other type of irritation, which has severe pain and considerable blood excreted.

Apply cupping on the arms, then take amber oil (one teaspoon) and a half cup of Betonite to stop the bleeding. Apply cupping on the bowels, below the navel, alternating right to left side. Keep up the cupping for four hours to stop the diarrhea.

13.3 Phlegm Coming from Intestines

The cause of irritation of the intestinal walls or a bursting of a ballooned part of the colon. Use herbal preparation: pomegranate skin, sumac, myrtle, and cooked white rice (in equal parts of a tablespoon each); boil them in eight ounces of water, add a teaspoon of limestone, and use as an enema.

13.4 Gripe

Generally a little moisture comes out with the stools; it may be mixed with a little blood. There is pain. There may be an obstruction of the bowels the body wants to expel, but it cannot do it by itself. The sign is that when the person eats melon and other dried seeds, they won't pass out through the bowels. Soften the intestines with warm drinks and enemas, and consult a physician. Never give astringents; this is sometimes fatal.

Phlegm, yellow, and black bile can also cause gripe. These remedies were given in 13.2.

Using enemas and suppositories is more helpful in intestinal ailments than drinking teas, as the enemas are able to go directly to the afflicted area.

If the gripe is caused by intense heat accumulating in the lower part of the intestine, the sign is feeling heavy palpitation; sometimes a fever arises, and there is difficulty in urinating.

Apply cupping just under the waist, above the pubic bone, and go on a moderate fast.

If the cause is an excess of cold temperament reaching to the rectum, the remedy is applying warm fomentations to the lower abdomen, rubbing cactus oil on the anus, and sitting on a "hot seat" (made by heating bricks and covering with a towel folded over several times—a hot water bottle works as well). If the anus and intestines are painful and sore on sitting down, just to rub with beeswax and egg yolk with rose oil added is enough.

13.5   Intestinal Pain from Gripe, Swelling, and Colic

If there is pain in the intestine without any of the causes mentioned in 13.4, the cause must be determined by a doctor. If the pain is felt after drinking laxative medicines, drinking warm water in large mouthfuls and rubbing the abdomen with rose oil is sufficient.

13.6   Gas and Grumbling of Intestines

If the cause is eating gas-producing foods or overeating, the remedy is to alter the diet and eating habits. Eat rose preserves and add four or five drops of pure rose water to tea several times a day. If the cause is coldness and weakness of the intestine, the sounds of grumbling in the intestine are there in spite of good foods in proper amounts. Remedy: Reduce the amount of food eaten at one sitting and add cayenne pepper as a condiment to foods.

13.7   About Colic

This is a severe pain felt in the intestine, accompanied by constipation, or very small hard stools passed with great difficulty. If the cause is excess of thick phlegm in the system, the signs are constipation and the tendency to desire sour and salty things. Soften the intestines with enemas and suppositories, and afterward give a laxative to cleanse the colon completely. Adding rice-bran syrup to the diet can help alleviate constipation, especially in children.

After the constipation is removed, do not consume food for twenty-four hours. The best food after this day-long fast is pea soup containing a little chicken meat. Partridge and young lamb are also good. Don't drink much water; instead, drink six ounces of rose water, anise water, or honey water. Eating naun (see recipe, Chapter 4) is also helpful.

Stomach-gas colic is caused by melancholy feelings, and the signs are that the pain happens very suddenly, even though there is no gas in the intestines or stomach. In another form, there is a great deal of sour belching but no pain. The black bile humour must be purged and a good body massage performed with oil. If there is swelling in the intestine, rub with rose oil and drink warm water.

13.8 Constipation without Pain

Remedy: Syrup of violet with almond oil, in equal parts of two tablespoons, to move bowels.

13.9 Intestinal Worms

There are four kinds of worms that infest the stomach or intestines. One is long; another is wide like pumpkin seeds; another is round; and another is very small, like vinegar worms. The signs of worms are that the lips are dry during the day and wet at night, and sometimes the person wakes with a little pool of saliva on the pillow. You may be able to see worms in the stool, but not always.

If the temperament is hot, which it is likely to be, never give hot medicine. The following mixture is said to kill the worms: Make an infusion of the skin of sour pomegranate and the roots, about an ounce of each, and drink a wineglassful twice a day. If the person cannot drink the liquid, use it as an enema. The best medicine for small worms is to make a suppository of henna and wax. Insert into the rectum, but leave a little part of the suppository exposed. After a day or less, take the suppository out; some of the small worms will be embedded in it. Olive oil is also good for any kind of worms; drink a tablespoon or rub it on the anus.

Colonic irrigation is also quite successful in washing worm infestations out of the intestines. The addition of oxygen to the irrigation is recommended, since the worms dwell in the intestines where there is little oxygen. This should be done only by a physician.

The Kidneys

General Considerations

The kidneys are paired organs, each located next to the spine along the back wall of the abdomen at about the level of the last thoracic vertebrae. The unit of the kidney composition and function is the *nephron,* about one million to each kidney.

The nephrons maintain the constancy of the blood by filtering and reabsorbing substances that are present in excess quantity and ejecting them as urine.

The secretion of urine is accomplished by direct nerve impulses on the blood vessels leading to the kidneys, by other nerve impulses acting on endocrine glands, and through the effects of pituitary and adrenal hormones.

14.1 Bad Temperament of the Kidneys

The sign is difficult or incomplete urination or other signs of hot or cold intemperament. The remedy is to inhale vapor of camphor; its essence travels to the kidneys. Do not inhale too much of this essence, as it can lead to loss of sex drive.

14.2 Emaciation of the Kidneys

The signs are white or colorless urine and pain, weakness of the body, loss of virility, backache, and headache. Remedy: Reinforce the kidneys by diet consisting of large amounts of pure water, kidney meats, parsley, leafy green vegetables, wheat germ, and fresh green peas. Avoid coffee, alcohol, and other stimulants.

14.3 Weakness of the Kidneys

Its signs are backache, especially when bowing, bending down, or turning from side to side; weakness of virility; and lessened tendency to urinate. Cure by diet as in 14.2 and the detoxification regimen. If the cause is bad temperament, adjust it.

The *hakims* say that excessive sexual intercourse will cause weakness of the kidneys, by causing the outlet of the kidneys to widen or slacken. Reinforce the kidneys by diet.

14.4 Gas of Kidney

Its sign is pain in the kidney area, but no intestinal flatulency and no heaviness. The pain diminishes as the time for eating approaches. Remedy: Make a pomade of common dill, cumin, wild rue, and dates (equal parts), and apply externally to the kidneys. Drink honey water with vinegar and eat foods that remove gas (see 13.6).

Fig. 10 • The Kidneys

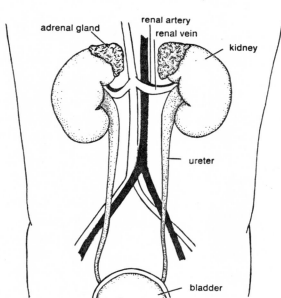

14.5 Kidney Ache

Its cause is gas, swelling, weakness, stone, or ulcer of the kidney. Remove the cause, consulting the appropriate sections, and afterward give this medicine: cooked dates (three ounces) and a quarter-ounce each of common dill and marshmallow made into a decoction; take a teaspoon three times a day.

14.6 Swelling of the Kidneys

The signs of this are the same as for swelling of the liver (10.7). Sometimes pain is felt in the waist. If swelling is in the right kidney, the pain is felt a little above the kidneys, close to the liver. If swelling is in the left kidney it is felt somewhat lower, because the right kidney is a little higher than the left one. If swelling is in the ducts of the kidneys, there is difficulty in passing urine. If the swelling is in the lower part of the kidney, in the intestinal area, the pain is entirely internal and creates colic. If the swelling is chronic, go on a detoxification program, and correct the diet by including more fresh greens and cutting back on fruits. No sugar.

14.7 Ulcers of the Kidneys

The sign is passing of phlegm, blood, and small bits of tissue with the urine, and there is pain in the kidneys. Adjust the phlegm humour, but do not give strong purgatives (mild ones are all right). After adjusting the phlegm humour, diuretics are advised. Wild cherry syrup is the herbal recommendation.

14.8 Dry Scabbing of the Kidneys

The symptom of this is itching in the area of the kidneys, and its remedy is to use a purgative. Use an emetic two times a week, and give syrup of violet. Drop two or three drops of sweet almond oil into the urethra outlet.

14.9 Kidney Stones

If the system is congested with toxins, this ailment may recur. Detoxification is recommended. The signs of a condition leading to kidney stones are heaviness of the stomach, extended abdomen, yellowness or redness of the urine, passing of small stones, and excruciating pain. The symptoms are most often severe. Adjust the digestion and avoid all stimulating foods and spices, eating very little. Refraining from sexual intercourse, sleeping on a plain cotton mattress, frequent mild baths, and drinking lots of cold water during meals and upon waking are all recommended to help prevent stone formation. Usually the pain is so severe during an attack of kidney stones that treatment by narcotics is employed. Consult a qualified physician.

The Urinary Bladder

General Considerations

The urinary bladder is an oval-shaped muscular sac located in the front part of the pelvic cavity, just behind the pubic area.

The bladder is a storage place for urine, which is received from the ureters, which open into the bladder on the lower back side of the bladder. The urine is discharged periodically through the urethra.

The ureters enter the bladder at an oblique angle, and there is a mucous membrane at each opening that acts as a valve.

The urethra is the duct that carries the urine from the bladder to outside the body. In men, it also carries the semen. In women, its function is solely excretory.

Urine consists of 95 percent water and 5 percent solids. The principal organic constituent of urine is urea (23 percent); the two chlorides, sodium chloride (9 percent) and potassium chloride (2.5 percent), make up the main inorganic substances.

Under normal conditions, urine has the following characteristics:

1. *Color:* amber, due to urochrome, a pigment of unknown origin. Drugs, illness, or certain foods may alter color.

2. *Transparency:* Normal urine is clear and transparent. It will become cloudy after standing for a while, due to bacterial action. Bacterial infection of the urogenital tract can produce similar cloudy urine.

3. *pH:* Urine is usually acid, with a pH around 6.0. This acidity is mainly due to the presence of sodium acid phosphate. The pH varies considerably with diet, with vegetable and fruit

diets lowering the acidity and resulting in alkaline urine. Acidity increases in certain diseases (such as diabetes), and varies throughout the day as elimination of wastes and toxins occurs.

15.1 Swelling of the Bladder

If the cause is hot intemperament, there is severe pain in the pubic area, with gas, hot fever, and difficulty in urinating. The remedy calls for cupping on the leg veins and weak diuretics. Do not use pomades. If the heat is causing putrefaction and accumulated matter, try to ripen the matter and purge it.

If the cause is from cold nature intemperament, the signs are hard swelling of the bladder and the signs of black bile and phlegm humour imbalance.

Remedy: For phlegm imbalance, vomiting, enemas, sitz baths, drinking diuretics, honey water, and decoction of cassia. In black bile humour imbalance, apply pomades made of laxative herbs (cucumber seeds, cassia, dates, anise, and the like, mixed with almond oil). Do not give too many diuretic herbs as it may cause too rapid detoxification, which can be known from a high alkaline pH of the urine.

15.2 Ulcers of the Bladder

The signs are small amounts of tissue passed with the urine, burning, and difficulty in urinating. The remedy is the same as for kidney ulcers (14.7). If there is also rheum coming out, dropping a tablespoon of distilled water mixed with half a teaspoon of honey into the urethra has been found useful. In urinary disease, applying the remedy via the urethral outlet with a sterile eyedropper is more helpful, as the herbs go directly to work. Women can apply herbs by douche injection.

15.3 Dry Scab of the Bladder

The signs are itching in the area of the bladder, pain, burning on urination, and blood secreted with the urine. The treatment should be designed more to adjust than to purge, because the adjustment has an immediate effect. This is the opposite of the treatment of kidney scab, in which purging is better and preferred. Put a few drops of this infusion into the urethra: equal parts of the mucilage of seeds of quince, mother's milk, and almond oil. It is always useful to use an enema in problems with the urinary bladder. The best foods are barley, oily soups, wheat germ, whole grains, green leafy vegetables, beans, and nuts. Avoid salt, coffee, and acid-forming foods as well as fruits.

15.4 Clotting of Blood in Bladder

When incomplete elimination of blood occurs, there may be clotting in the bladder itself. The signs that this has happened are fainting and both sides of the body becoming cold. There may be general trembling of the body, especially after a blow or other injury. Strong diuretics should be given, along with cooked black-eyed peas and wild rue tea. Dropping ash of fig tree in the urethra is useful as well. The diet can be amended to include chicken soup with black-eyed peas and cinnamon. Bleeding from the urethra after a wound requires medical treatment as soon as possible.

15.5 Ache of Urinary Bladder

The cause can be either swelling, ulcer, or dry scab of the bladder. These were all discussed in earlier sections. There are two other causes to be explained.

1. Ache caused by bad temperament. If the temperament is too hot, the person feels thirsty and there is a burning sensation on urination. The remedy is to adjust the diet with cold-natured foods and to use pomades of cold herbs. If the cause is cold nature intemperament, the sign is whiteness or colorlessness of the urine. The remedy involves keeping the person warm under blankets, pouring warm water over the urinary bladder, and improving the diet.

2. Ache due to effort of bladder to repulse effete matter. The sign is the appearance of putrid matter with the urine. Drink plenty of water to help the elimination process.

15.6 Displacement of the Bladder

The cause may be congenital or due to a fall, severe beating, or blows to the back. An internal surgeon should be consulted for congenital defects as soon as they are suspected. Otherwise, give sweet basil and sweetmeats. If the displacement lingers, imprisonment of urine may occur. Consult a physician.

15.7 Flatulency of Urinary Bladder

The sign is the physical appearance of distention of the bladder over the pubic bone. If there is heaviness of the bladder with the area of distention moving from one place to another, the cause is only trapped air. But if there is heaviness without transference of the distention, the cause is moisture being mixed with the trapped air.

Remedy: Give a decoction of peppermint roots with a teaspoon of castor oil added to it for a few days. Then give two ounces of castor oil every few hours, and rub the bladder area with saffron oil. If there is trouble urinating, dry and pulverize the skin of a yellow melon and give a teaspoon of it every few hours. If there is moisture mixed with the trapped air, emetics are recommended. Marijuana, tea, and figs are recommended, singly or together.

15.8 Stones of Urinary Bladder

The sign of presence of stones in the bladder is that immediately after emptying the bladder, the person desires to urinate again. In men, there may be a sudden erection without stimulation, which may remain for some time, but there is no pain in the bladder unless it is blocked by a stone. It is rather common that stones are formed in the bladder or pass down from the kidneys into the bladder for expulsion. A sharp pain in the area of the kidneys and back of the thighs, which then passes, is a sign that a stone is descending from the kidneys into the bladder. The remedy was given in 14.9. Surgical removal of stones may be necessary, so consult a physician if the signs persist and are severe.

If the stone is stopped in the outlet of the bladder and there is much pain and inability to urinate, a recommended first aid measure is to have the person lie on his back, lift the legs, pour warm water on the pubic bone, and apply vigorous massage from the chest down to the pubic bone. This may dislodge the stone and allow it to pass out.

15.9 *Burning on Urination*

If caused by dry scab of the kidney or bladder, consult 14.8 and 15.3. It may also be caused by an ulcer in the outlet of the penis, which is discussed later. The cause may also be due to liver heat or prevalence of biliousness, which signs are discussed in Chapter 6. Apply what was given in 10.1. If adjustment is not sufficient, use enemas and drop three or four drops of this mixture into the urethra: mother's milk, one ounce; rose oil and almond oil, half an ounce each. Males should soak the penis in alkaline water; females bathe the urethra opening with same. Make alkaline water by soaking three figs in a pint of water and straining.

15.10 *Retention of Urine*

Causes for which remedies have already been mentioned are swelling of kidney (14.6), swelling of urinary bladder (15.1), urinary or kidney stones (14.9, 15.8), rheum in the bladder (15.1), or gas of the bladder (15.7, 20.19). Retention of urine may also be caused by ulcers or boils in the bladder (see 15.2).

Retention may also be caused by internal growths on the bladder outlet or congenital smallness or other change in the outlet. The sign of congenital defects is that there are no other signs of disease; the only remedy is surgical correction.

Slackness of the muscles of the bladder is another case; this is the problem if urine is forced out when one presses on the bladder from above the pubic bone. Treat this by giving warm drinks and teas; consult the section on paralysis (2.20) for oils to rub on the bladder area.

If the cause is obstruction of the vessel between the bladder and urethra by phlegm, the sign is a sensation of heaviness in the area of the pubis. Remedy: Give strong diuretics and have the person sit in warm water. If the cause is weakness of the expulsive power of the bladder, the sign is that the person can delay going to the bathroom for several hours, but when he does go, the urine will not come out. Remedy: Have him sit in warm water and press the bladder to expel the urine. To revive the expulsive power of the bladder, apply a salve of red clover on the pubis. If this doesn't work, the urine will have to be extracted with a catheter, which requires the assistance of a medical doctor.

Another cause of inability to urinate is constipation and dryness occurring in the bladder outlet, due to severe heat. The signs are heat patches over the pubis, an improved sense of well-being after drinking fluids, and inability to expel small amounts of urine (i.e., the person can only urinate after a long period). The remedy is to give moistening and cold drinks.

If the cause is weakness of the urinary urge, the remedy is dropping several drops of saffron oil into the urethra, applying sweet-smelling pomades, and drinking lots of water and moderate doses of castor oil.

15.11 Involuntary Expulsion of Urine

If the cause is slackness of the bladder muscles, hot intemperament, or swelling of an adjacent part, the remedies are given in 15.10. Involuntary urination may also come from taking too many diuretics, consuming too much melon, and so forth. Remove the cause.

This can also be caused by misalignment of the lumbar vertebrae after a fall or a blow to the back or urinary bladder. This needs correction by a physician. If the blow has caused improper alignment of the vertebrae toward the inside (anterior), apply cupping to the vertebrae affected. If it is toward the outside (posterior), you can probably notice the specific vertebrae out of alignment by having the person remove his clothes and bend from the waist. Have the person lie on his stomach. Put the palms of both hands on either side of the spinal column and give a downward motion to correct the spine. NOTE: It is best to see a chiropractor, osteopath, naprapath, or similar practitioner. However, many masseurs can correct this as well.

If the expulsion of urine is the result of nerve damage, there is no herbal cure. Consult a physician.

15.12 Bedwetting

Although some adults are afflicted with urinating in bed, it is mainly a problem with children. (Consult 15.10 about slackness of the bladder muscles.) Do not give any food or water for two hours before bedtime. If the child begins to urinate during sleep, try to wake him up and take him to the bathroom. This medicine is advised: cumin, mastic, myrtle, a quarter-ounce each; mix with three or four ounces of honey and give in teaspoon doses morning and evening.

15.13 Urine Mixed with Blood

If there is no pain or mucous, it may be due to irritation of the nerves of the kidney. If the blood is coming in small amounts regularly, this is probably the cause. While any bleeding needs attention by a physician, you can apply first aid if necessary to stop the bleeding by cupping over the bladder, pouring cold water over the pubis, and giving a medicine of jujube syrup with coriander.

If weakness of the kidneys is causing bleeding, the urine looks white and thick; if it is caused in the liver, the urine is reddish and thin. In either case, the kidneys and liver must be reinforced.

The Male
Reproductive System

For the purposes of the following sections, these descriptions of tissue are given: the skin of the abdomen is called the *hypochondria;* the layer under it is called the *peritoneum;* and the fatty layer under the peritoneum which is touching the intestines is called the *omentum.*

16.1 Weakness of Virility

Completeness of the sex drive depends upon the health of the male organs. A lack of virility appears in two syndromes; one is that the libido and drive for sexual intercourse are weak, the other is that an erection is difficult to achieve and maintain.

Weakness of sex drive The first cause is eating too little food. Since the body depends on food to sustain life, the spirit, humours, and blood that are the substances of sexual energy diminish. The signs of this condition are general weakness, loss of energy, and feeling hungry much of the time. The remedy is to consume more nutritious food and stimulating herbs such as spearmint, and to remove anxiety and worry so that life may be enjoyed. Listening to music is recommended.

A second sign of weakened sex drive is that there is reduced semen production in spite of proper nutrition. The sign is emission of very small amounts of semen during intercourse. The cause of this is bad temperament in the semen-producing organs.

There is a difference between insufficient semen production and low sperm count—they can occur quite independently of each other. Also, low sperm count can be caused by excessive exposure to radiation and certain chemicals, not uncommon hazards for American workers.

A third sign of weakened sex drive is that even though semen is produced in sufficient quantity, it is not emitted during ejaculation. If this is the case, there is emission of only clear fluid, and the semen is retained or it comes out very thick and with difficulty. Also, during sexual foreplay, the penis is semi-flaccid but becomes erect during intercourse. The remedy is to eat humorally hot foods and drink teas made from hot herbs.

Fourth, abstention from intercourse for an extended period will cause the sex drive to become weak. The mind must convey to the body a willingness to perform sex; this can be stimulated by observing animals performing intercourse and discussions about people engaged in intercourse. Pellitory root rubbed in cottonseed oil applied to the pubis and penis is also recommended.

Fifth, loss of sex drive can be due to feelings of inferiority or an imagination that the male is incapable of performing sex adequately. The man gradually loses all interest, even though

Fig. 11 • The Male Reproductive Organs

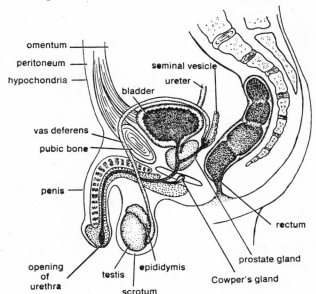

he may be young and healthy and be producing plenty of semen. This must be treated by personal guidance and counseling.

The sex drive may also become weak due to related weakness of the heart, kidney, liver, or brain. Consult the section on these organs for removal of these conditions.

16.2   Slackness of Penis

The first cause is from weakness of the sex drive or abstinence from sex for a long period. In the case of abstinence from sex, washing the penis with warm water before intercourse is helpful, as is massaging the penis with oil of musk or ambergris.

The cause may be due to lack of production of the humours in the lower part of the body, and is caused by imbalance of heat, cold, or moisture.

The nerves governing the erective faculty may become blunted due to congestion of phlegm or exposure to extreme coldness, for which the signs are the thinness of the seminal fluid and that it "leaks" when there is no sexual stimulation. Seek the remedy in the section on paralysis (2.20). Using an enema and suppositories for increasing heat and removing phlegm congestion are useful. (The *hakims* say that the one whose penis does not shrink when placed in cold water cannot be cured.) Some of the remedies to stimulate full erection are washing the penis with an infusion of celery seeds and rubbing with oil of purslane. Oil of lily-of-the-valley is said to have the same effect.

16.3   Premature Ejaculation

One of the causes is lack of self-control. The signs of this are whiteness and thinness of the semen; the remedy is purging the system with medicine for cold intemperament and taking an emetic.

Another cause is prevalence of semen and blood, which is shown by very hard and strong erections and engorgement of the glans with blood. One remedy is to increase frequency of intercourse and to eat less food, making the diet consist of more sour things and foods that decrease production of blood. If the semen is expelled with excessive force, there is burning on ejaculation and the semen is thin and yellow. Decoction of lettuce seeds and other cold-natured medicines are recommended. Hasty discharge may also be caused by weakness of the sex organs, which need to be strengthened according to 16.1.

16.4 Excessive Sex Drive

The man seems tied to his emotions and can't seem to get sex off his mind. The first cause is prevalence of semen and blood, which is known by flushed cheeks, rash on the chest, and similar signs of heat. Using laxatives and eating sour foods may help to decrease the urge. If the semen is expelled with great force, drinking honey with ice water is helpful.

There may be adequate semen but general weakness and insufficiency of blood, whose signs are excess discharge of thin and white semen and much flatulence. Remedy: Give wild rue seed and fennel seed, each a quarter-gram, with ten drops of oil of almond added, a teaspoon with tea twice a day.

Another cause of excessive sex drive is due to strength of the semen-producing organs but weakness of other important organs of the body, such as strong sperm production but weakness of the heart. The remedy is to stem the sexual energy by wholesome exercise, building up the other systems of the body.

The sex drive may be increased along with appearance of boils, ulceration, or itching of the penis outlet. The sign is primarily excessive lust and intercourse. If the boils turn into ulcers, there will be pain. The remedy is to use the purgative for the urinary bladder, given in 14.7 and 15.2.

If excessive sex drive is due to prevalence of the production of gas in the body, the sign is intense erection, for which cold-natured herbs should be given as tea several times per day. If black bile humoral inharmony signs are present, give a black bile diuretic as well.

16.5   Corrupted Semen

There are two kinds: (1) a moist substance comes out, although it is emitted not from the seminal vesicles but from another duct above the seminal vessel; (2) a sticky moisture is expelled with the urine.

The cause of either of these may be prevalence of semen or slackness of the veins serving the seminal or semen-producing organs. The remedy is given in 16.3. A second cause of corrupted semen is convulsion of the muscle of the seminal vein, which is known from expulsion of semen at the first period of erection, or successive erection and loss of erection of the penis. The remedy is rubbing rose or other mild oil on the penis and testicles, and curing the convulsion.

Corrupted semen is also caused by weakness of the kidneys, or can be due to a condition following rapid weight loss. The sign is that after intercourse, a white thick substance similar to semen comes out with the urine. Apply what was said about weakness of the kidney in 14.3.

If semen is spontaneously emitted when a man hears others talking about sex or when he himself is thinking about engaging in sex, he should try to develop more self-control.

16.6   Excretion of Blood with Semen

The cause is weakness of the kidneys and testicles. Soak the testicles in a bowl of mastic with some plain oil added, and strengthen the kidneys (see 14.2).

16.7   Constant Erection of the Penis

If the cause is prevalence of blood, adjust the blood humour, use blood purgative, and eat cold foods and herbal teas. If the temperament is cold and dry, procure emesis and give medicine to remove flatulency. Afterward, rub oil of wild rue on the pubis, genitals, and back.

16.8 Defecation during Ejaculation

The cause is excess moisture and weakness of the sexual organs
and bowel muscles. Reinforce the bowel and abdominal muscles
with exercise such as sit-ups, and use this suppository: false
acacia (locust-tree leaves), pomegranate flowers, gum Arabic
(or mastic), equal parts. Rub the anus with oil of hyacinth.
Immediately before intercourse, the stomach should be empty.

16.9 Feeling of Itch in Intestine

This comes with the urge to have intercourse with a woman,
and can be caused by foul substances eaten (remedy: purgative)
or prevalence of improper temperament (remedy: eat sour
foods).

16.10 Swelling of the Testicles

If the cause is in the blood humour, the sign is heaviness,
swelling, and heat of testicles. If the cause is biliousness, the
sign is very intense heat of the testicles. Apply cupping on the
back and legs, and afterward use rose oil. (Consult the sections
on general swellings.)

If the cause is imbalance of the phlegm humour, the testicles
look pale and white. The remedy for phlegm imbalance is first
to cause vomiting, then give cooked anise seeds, licorice-root
tea, rose preserve, and diuretics for phlegm. Use a salve of
equal parts of green beans and peas (dried, pounded, and
sifted) and honey.

If the cause is black bile humour, the testicles are swollen
and hard. Give the diuretic for black bile.

If the cause of testicle swelling is flatulency, the testicles seem
full and inflated. The remedy is to apply a cloth soaked with
decoction made from gas-reducing herbs such as peppermint,
catnip, or camomile. If that doesn't work, try vomiting and
using diuretics; vomiting is most recommended for conditions
affecting the lower parts of the body.

NOTE: If the origin of the swelling is in the skin of the

testicles, the symptoms can be felt mildly. If the cause is in the testicles themselves, the symptoms are more severe, and there is often feverishness and thirst.

16.11 Enlarged Testicles

The cause may be fatty tissue, not swelling. Make a salve of hemlock bark and infusion of coriander, and add a little vinegar to it. This can be used as an application to the testicles, or to the breasts if they are swollen. Fasting is required.

16.12 Convulsion of the Penis

The sign is shrinking or twisting up of the penis. The remedy is using a purgative, purifying the blood humour, and afterward using a purgative again. Correct the diet.

16.13 Aching Testicles

The cause may be swelling (16.10). It may also be due to accumulated gas from sexual excitement that is not gratified for an extended period. Fomentations and lubrication with olive or rose oil are usually sufficient, along with keeping a little warmer than usual. If the cause is injury to the testicles from a blow, apply a salve made of violet, marshmallow, pumpkin, water lily (white or yellow), equal parts. Add some crushed seeds of marijuana if available.

16.14 Shrinking of Testicles

The cause is exposure to cold. Take a warm bath to restore elasticity of skin.

16.15 Ascended Testicles

The testicles sometimes ascend into the hypochondria, the soft part just under the cartilage of the pubic bone, and cannot be seen. When this happens, there is difficulty in urinating. If they ascend only slightly (as at time of ejaculation), it is not harmful nor painful, but if they remain up for a long time, it is harmful. The remedy is to sit in a warm bath, rub oil of euphorbium herb on the testicles and let it be absorbed. Cupping can be applied to the testicles if bathing does not cause descension.

NOTE: Sometimes the penis recedes back into the body cavity. The same measures can be applied.

16.16   Drooping Testicles

The veins of the testicles become elongated so that the testicles hang down farther than they should. The remedy is in the section on veins of the leg (18.5). If the skin of the testicles becomes hardened, apply the remedy in 16.10.

16.17   Slackness of Testicle Skin

Use a remedy composed of myrtle, rose, and pomegranate flower. Make a salve or a weak decoction and bathe the testicles in it.

16.18   Ulcers of Penis and Testicles and Genital Area

One kind of ulceration is fresh, appearing suddenly. Use a purgative and detoxify. Another kind develops slowly and lingers. This remedy is recommended: dragon's-blood and myrrh, each a half gram; juice of aloe vera and resin, 2 drams. Make a salve, mix with an ounce of rose oil, and apply.

NOTE: The sign of a penis ulcer in the urethra is burning on urination and pain. The remedy for this is given in 15.2.

16.19   Swelling of the Penis

See the remedy in 16.10.

16.20   Hard Boils Appearing on the Penis

Mix half an ounce of fennel seed in two ounces of vinegar, add a little vegetable oil, and apply to boils.

16.21 Obstruction of the Urethra

If the cause is boils, the urine is expelled with great difficulty, and burning is felt. Rub decoction of purslane and melon seeds mixed with violet oil and almond oil on the penis several times per day. When the boil opens and begins to drain, drop a few drops of mother's milk and violet oil into the opening.

If the urethra is sticking together from secretions from the boil, the urine comes out with difficulty but without pain. Drink a mixture made of equal parts of cooked dates, sweet melilot, common mugwort, and sweet marjoram. A little of this can be poured through a fine strainer and dropped into the opening of the penis.

16.22 Twisting of the Penis

This is caused either by swelling of the muscle of the penis or convulsion of the nerves in the penis. Rubbing the penis with warm oils and taking a warm bath during which the penis can be straightened are recommended.

16.23 Separation of the Peritoneum

Separation of the peritoneum occurs on the inner side of the thigh, toward the testicles. When there is a separation of this tissue, adjacent parts of the omentum or intestines (and sometimes fluids) come down into the testicles. This condition is called *cornia* in natural medicine. It has four forms:

1. Water descends little by little, with gurgling, grumbling and other sounds. Sometimes it is accompanied by spastic pains like colic. The remedy is to rub the area slowly and massage the intestine. Pouring warm water on it also helps, as does sitting in warm baths. Then, put a poultice on the testicles, also covering the inner part of the groin and pubic area. The poultice is made as follows: pound equal parts of pine buds, resin (or gum), mastic, false acacia, pomegranate flowers, dragon's-blood, aloe gum, juniper berries, and seaweed. Mix in enough turtle oil to give consistency (water will do as well), and spread on a cloth. Bind in place for three days and keep

the person lying on his back. After three days, he can get up and move around carefully. Add much cumin seed to the food.

2. Gas moving around in the groin, with severe grumbling. Eat no gas-producing foods and make a binding of clean cloth that holds the area firmly in place.

3. The testicles become full of fluid and heavy. The remedy is to remove the water or liquid by applying what was said about dropsy in 10.14.

4. Thickness, hardness, and stretching of the testicles. This is different from simple swelling of the testicles in that the latter is caused by a corrupted substance. Purge the black bile humour and apply what was said in 16.10.

16.24 Hernia of the Abdomen Hypochondria (and Hernia of the Groin)

It sometimes occurs that the peritoneum tissue is torn close to the area of the navel, or higher, even though the hypochondria itself is sound. Thus, what is situated below the peritoneum is distended and lifts up the hypochondria. Sometimes it happens that in the area of the groin, a break appears in the peritoneum, also causing hernia. The only procedure that can be recommended by natural medicine is to apply heavy binding. Surgery may be necessary to repair the tears in the wall of the peritoneum. Consult a medical doctor for advice and examination.

16.25 Changes in the Navel

Infrequently, due to improper cutting of the umbilical cord at birth, various changes occur in the navel scar. If it becomes protruded, it can be repaired while the infant is still a few weeks old. When it becomes healed and scar tissue forms, it is more difficult to repair.

Changes at times other than infancy may indicate herniation of the peritoneum wall, discussed in the preceding section.

Other changes can be caused by excess phlegm moisture gathering in the area of the navel (as in dropsy), gathering of excess flatulence, growth of excess flesh in the navel, or blood accumulating under the navel due to a rupture of a blood vessel.

The sign of a hernia is the turning inward of the fleshy part of the navel, with or without intestinal sounds. The sign of accumulated moisture of phlegm is heaviness in the navel area, and the sign of flatulence is extreme softness of the navel.

The remedy for flatulence is mentioned in 10.14. Extraneous growth of flesh must be treated by a physician, as must signs of broken blood vessels. An emergency salve of wax and rose oil can be applied until a doctor can treat it.

The Female Reproductive System

17.1 *Suppressed Menses*

A mild diuretic is recommended, as follows: take 2 drams of half-pounded anise, boil in a cup of water for five minutes. Filter, and add one-half dram each of powdered cucumber seeds and melon seeds. Sweeten with honey and drink.

The specific emmenagogue to open the menstrual flow is composed of cassia and fennel seed, 8 grams each; castoreum and juniper berries, 2 grams each. Take 4 to 8 grains every morning, followed by 40 grams of anise tea. This will open the menstrual flow if the cause is not due to high temperature and insufficient blood.

A medicine to open the menstrual flow or suppressed semen is composed of fennel seed, wild rue, wormwood, and celery seeds, 2 grams each; 5 figs, rose hips, and honey, combined to make 40 grams. Boil together for five minutes and consume in tablespoon doses twice a day for three days. Stop for three days, then repeat dose for three more days.

17.2 *Excessive Menstrual Flow*

The prevalence of menstrual blood is easily noticed. The remedy is to decrease the blood by using enemas and cupping on the abdomen. If the blood is thin, the cause is biliousness, for which the remedy is enemas, thickening of blood, suppositories, and rubbing sandalwood on the pubis

If the cause is phlegm, there will be excessive blood, its character being white and thin. The remedy is decreasing the blood temperament. If the cause is excess of black bile, the remedy is to use a laxative to purge the black bile humour.

If the cause is hemorrhoids or ulcer of the womb, consult those sections.

At the time of rupture of the hymen, there may be blood flow. This can be remedied by sitting in astringent baths and rubbing the vulva with flower oils.

17.3 Vaginal Secretions

This is perhaps the most common nonspecific female complaint. While there may be bacterial infestation in some cases, the origin of most secretions is in imbalance of the medium of the vagina. It must be corrected according to general dietary regimen, using purgatives, and adjustment of either hot or cold intemperament (see beginning of Formulary).

Proper circulation of air is important; nylon underwear, girdles, leotards, and tights can cause or aggravate many minor

Fig. 12 • The Female Reproductive Organs

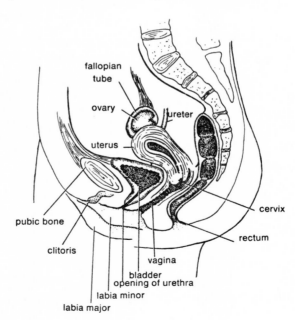

vaginal irritations. Cotton underwear "breathes" and allows better circulation.

NOTE: A seminal-like fluid can come from women too. The corruption and conditions of such emissions are the same as those for men, when related to general organ imbalance. Unusual discharge of female sexual fluids (copious discharge of Bartholin glands and excessive wetness of vagina) may be due to slackness of the mouth of the womb. The remedy is to procure emesis and bathe in astringent waters. The best medicine for slackness of the mouth of the womb is fennel seed, 3 drams, and root of lily-of-the-valley, 2 drams; add to pomegranate flower and rose hips, one-half dram each. Pound and sift, and give 2 drams with buttermilk or a glass of juiced green grapes.

17.4 Itching of the Vagina

To relieve this irritation, the remedy is made as follows: pound and sift equal parts of pennyroyal leaves, skin of pomegranate, and lentils. Mix with half a cup of vinegar or water. Spread on a thin piece of sterile cloth, a piece of cotton, or a commercial tampon, adding oil of violet and oil of rose. Insert in vagina to relieve vulva itching.

17.5 Contraception

Since the traditional cultures of the East prohibit abortion and generally have a positive desire to have large families, the concentration is more upon finding methods to aid conception than vice versa. There are valid physical and mental reasons for men and women to limit the growth of their families. The traditional midwives (*dais*) recommend that the women eat mung beans (*dahl*) and the seeds and flowers of acacia (acacia is an ingredient in several contraceptive jellies). Also recommended is having the woman jump up and down eight or nine times after intercourse, to cause the seminal fluid to fall down from the mouth of the womb. Rubbing the head of the penis with sesame oil is also recommended prior to intercourse.

17.6   False Pregnancy

All of the signs of pregnancy—swollen and tender breasts, absence of menstrual period, even the psychological feeling of being a mother—may appear even though conception has not occurred. The physical causes of the signs of pregnancy are dropsy, hard swelling of the womb, and ovarian cyst; fertilization of the ovum while in the fallopian tube is also considered a false pregnancy. Consult the sections dealing with these signs, if they are present.

17.7   About Inability to Conceive

The first cause is either hot, cold, dry, or moist intemperament of the womb. The sign of heat is that the blood expelled during the menstrual period is thick and tending to a blackish color. The sign of cold is scantiness of the menstrual flow and its coming late. The sign of dryness is lack of normal secretions of the vagina, including suppressed menses. The sign of moisture is vaginal discharge and excessive menstrual flow.

With a humoral intemperament, the woman may become pregnant, but the fetus usually does not survive beyond the third month.

Another cause of inability to conceive is obesity, and the remedy is to engage in a program of weight loss to bring the body to a normal weight range. Extreme thinness can also impair conception, and the woman must develop a more efficient metabolism by diet. The following are other imbalances that can prevent conception, along with the corrective measures for each:

Flatulence of womb   The signs of this are flatulence of the pubic area and of the vulva, which is noted by the emission of sounds of flatulence during intercourse; or, when you tap over the pubic bone, there is a hollow sound. The remedy is to remove the flatulence by taking 3 drams of castor oil with a tablespoon of cod liver oil every day, and adding fowl to the diet.

Deviation of mouth of womb The lack of proper alignment of internal female parts can cause the semen to be unable to flow into the womb for fertilization. Altering the positions of intercourse and avoiding any quick motions (such as standing up) directly after intercourse are advised.

Injuries to the womb and other conditions may cause inability to conceive. You should make certain that there are no underlying physical conditions before deciding that it is or is not possible to conceive.

Catnip for conception In Afghanistan, the most frequent recommendation to women who desire to conceive was to drink catnip tea several times per day. Other preparations for pregnancy induction include eating ground almonds and a tea made from a teaspoonful of spearmint, three teaspoons of cardamom seeds, a half teaspoonful of ground ginger, and a half teaspoonful each of ground walnuts and pistachios.

One of the problems of applying the remedies of the East to women in the West is that, according to the *dais,* the time conception is most likely to occur is considered to be the days immediately before, during, and after the menstrual period; this is the opposite of the schedule figured out by Western science.

A lack of conception sometimes is due to the male. Thus, the man should be considered in all aspects of his health to find out if there is any physical basis (infertile sperm, for example) for the inability of the couple to conceive *together.* Just as some fruits are unable to fertilize, some men and women are infertile from birth. The method used by the *hakims* as a preliminary determination of whether or not the man is infertile is to place his semen in water. If it floats, it is suspected to be impotent.

17.8 Frequent Miscarriage

The cause may be psychological or physical. The underlying conditions must be determined and removed. A decoction of tea of false unicorn is the best herbal preparation.

17.9 Difficult Birth

The traditional midwives advise women who have difficult births to drink raw goat's milk, as much as they can comfortably consume and digest, from the eighth month of pregnancy. When the time for birth is near, she should avoid cold water, vinegar, and all cold foods. The attendant at the birth should rub sweet almond oil with oil of linseed, half-warmed, on the mouth of the womb to facilitate birth. The specific medicine recommended in the healers' text for delivery is the following: ground cinnamon, and cassia, 4 grams each; cooked with syrup of violet or pea water, in tablespoon doses. The mother should not smell perfumes at the time of birth.

There are now many groups of midwives operating in the United States, and their number is growing rapidly. Most of the magazines on natural medicine have articles on natural childbirth, and with a little inquiring, you can find someone to provide you with the names of natural practitioners who will deliver at home under natural conditions. It is perfectly legal for a father to deliver his own child, but you should have an expert medical person available as backup in case there are complications in the delivery. There is no time whatsoever to learn during the delivery itself, and if you are planning to deliver your own child at home, the best course would be to have a general education about the procedures and techniques to be employed. The books at the end of Chapter 6 can be a beginning. Women with kidney disease, high blood pressure, and other abnormal conditions are high-risk mothers who should probably consider hospital births.

17.10 Imprisonment of the Chorion and Death of Fetus

The chorion is the outermost membrane covering the fetus. The signs that the death of the fetus has occurred are that there is no heartbeat, no movement, and the hands of the mother are cold and the pulse is erratic. Of course, removal of a fetus is a procedure for a medical doctor. If none is available, the medicine advised is to boil 3 drams each of musk, maidenhair herb, and juniper berries; add 2 drams of pennyroyal and drink with several tablespoons of sugar. After consuming this, make the mother sneeze by sniffing black pepper and crushed fennel seed. When she is about to sneeze, cover tightly the nose and mouth, to transfer the force of the expulsion inward. If no medicines work, the fetus must be separated from the umbilicus and removed, which requires someone trained to do so.

17.11   Imprisonment of the Afterbirth

The advice is the same as given for suppressed menses. The remedy to relieve the back pains sometimes felt after birth is to make a decoction of linseed and bathe the womb with it (malva flowers are also recommended).

17.12   Insufficiency of Milk

The breast has the capacity to convert blood into milk, just as the testicles convert blood into semen. Insufficiency of milk has three causes.

1. *Insufficiency of Blood.* This may be due to blood loss during delivery or the effects of chronic conditions. Give foods to increase blood, such as milk, egg yolks, and protein foods.

2. *Corruption of Blood due to Bad Temperament.* This must be corrected according to the directions in the beginning of the Formulary.

3. *Excess of Blood.* This means that the breast cannot "digest" the blood and make milk from it, due to the oversupply of blood itself. Apply cupping to the breasts.

Thinness, yellowness, and sharp smell of milk are due to biliousness. Intense whiteness, thickness, and sourness of milk are due to phlegm. Intense thickness, whiteness, and insufficiency of milk are due to black bile humour imbalance. A salty taste of milk is caused by mixing of phlegm with yellow bile. These must be corrected according to the humour affected.

17.13   Excess of Milk

The causes are the opposite of insufficiency of milk. To attempt to diminish the milk, use the remedies that open the menstrual flow. A half-ounce of cumin cooked in a pint of vinegar and rubbed on the breasts is used. In cases of cold intemperament, make a salve of wild rue (leaves and seeds) and seeds of beet for the breasts.

17.14 Swellings and Stretching of the Breast

This is due to either hot or cold intemperament of the breasts. For hot intemperament, make a salve of vinegar and cucumber. For cold intemperament, make a salve of pounded celery (or feverfew) and mix with anise water and apply to breasts.

17.15 Cessation of Milk Flow

If there is an excess of heat that makes the milk thick, there will be swelling of the breast. Excess of cold and obstruction of the flow will cause the same problem. The remedy is to remove the cause, consulting the sections on hot or cold intemperament and swellings. If the milk does not come out at first when the baby begins sucking, pour a little warm water over the breast, or "milk" the nipple slowly until the flow begins. It is felt that if a nursing mother is exposed to great fright, her milk flow may stop or become lessened.

If the interruption of flow causes infection, the signs are a change in the milk color, swelling, and foul taste of the milk. The infection must be ripened with a salve of linseed, marshmallow, and fennel seed. Mix in equal portions. Pound and sift. Mix with beet juice or water and apply as a salve to the breast two to three times per day. If the infection develops into an abscess, it will have to be treated by a doctor.

17.16 Bruising of the Breast

Make a salve by mixing the woman's own urine with olive oil, and apply to the breast. Apply cocoa butter to nipples if the baby makes them raw from sucking or chewing.

17.17   Pregnancy Tea

My wife spent the first eight months of her pregnancy in Afghanistan, and ate no foods containing any additives of any kind except for what Nature placed in them. She did not smoke and took no drugs of any kind. For the final month of her pregnancy, she began drinking herbal teas, which she felt were of benefit during the last stages of pregnancy and delivery. The teas she used were as follows:

> Squaw vine, spikenard, and raspberry, half a teaspoon each to make one and one-half cups of tea. Consumed twice daily during ninth month. Peppermint was added for taste and to alleviate nausea. At the first sign of labor, at the mildest pains, she made up a quart of blue cohosh, which was consumed for the remainder of the day. Her labor began at 1:30 P.M., approximately two hours after her "bag of waters" broke. She remained active and comfortable until 6:45 P.M., when she decided to lie down and begin the labor of delivery. An hour later the baby was born, without the use of any drugs, stimulants, or pain-relieving narcotics of any kind, other than Nature's herbs.

17.18   Ulcers and Wounds of the Womb

The sign is a feeling of pain and excretion of rheum or blood or both. In general, there can be no ulcer without the presence of rheum. The remedy is applied by douching the womb with rose oil, violet oil, and sugar water to cleanse the rheum. Then take a rectal enema with rose oil added (2 ounces to a pint of pure water, warmed). If the ulcer is in the neck of the womb, there is no need to use a douche; instead, apply to a tampon honey or boiled mother's milk and use as a vaginal suppository. This is very useful to purge the womb. If there is pain in the womb, add a little saffron (one grain) to the tampon mixture.

17.19   Hemorrhoids of the Womb

These are similar to hemorrhoids of the anus, and the remedy is the same as in 12.1 and 12.2.

17.20 Boils of the Womb

If the boils are in the neck of the womb, use an enema. Boils
can usually be felt by inserting the finger into the vagina. The
remedy is to adjust any intemperament and apply rose oil.

17.21 Protrusion of the Womb

This causes great pain in the pubis, anus, and groin. Trembling
of the body is often present, and the distension of soft tissue
can be felt in the vulva. First, purge the stomach and urinary
bladder by giving diuretics. Then take ten drops each of saffron
oil and water-lily oil with some musk oil or ambergris, and
apply half-warmed to the womb. Then, on some soft sterile
cloth, put an astringent such as false acacia (finely ground) and
musk and, while the woman is lying on her back, insert the
cloth. Leave the cloth in the womb this way for three days. Also
apply astringents on the pubis and vulva area, and apply
cupping on the waist close to the navel. The woman should
have perfumes to smell constantly. On the fourth day, renew
the soaked cloth.

Surgical correction is possible for this condition, and a
medical doctor should be consulted in every case.

17.22 Inclination of the Womb to One Side

This can be felt by the inserted fingers. There is pain on
intercourse. It causes dysentery and constipation. Have the
woman sit in a tub of warm water and afterward massage the
body with oil of feverfew. If there is excess moisture in the
womb, use an enema. If this course fails, a nurse or midwife
may be able to correct it with her fingers.

17.23 Swelling of the Womb

If the cause is hot substances or hot imtemperament, the signs
are fever, elevated pulse, bad digestion, and pain in the pubis
and groin. If the swelling occurs on both sides of the womb,
the remedy is the same as given for swelling of the urinary

bladder in 15.1. The swelling may run rheum and ulcers may form, which must be treated according to 17.18. If the cause is imbalance of the phlegm humour, the pubic area is very painful (remedy in 15.1). If the cause is imbalance of the black bile humour, the signs are hardness of the womb, inclination to one side, and little pain but prevalent heaviness of the womb. Use the black bile purgative, laxatives, and oils for massaging the pubis. Also, bathing twice a day in water of cooked marshmallow and common dill is useful.

17.24   Enlarged Swelling of the Womb

When there is a swelling that has ripened but has not "pierced," it is called enlarged swelling. If it is in the mouth of the womb, the swelling can be pierced mechanically by a physician. If the swelling is deep in the womb, give diuretics. Boil figs and mustard seeds (about one part figs to one-half part seed by volume) in one quart water. Strain off the sediment and use the water for a douche. Use the sediment remaining as a pomade to the pubis. After the swelling comes to a head and bursts, use the remedy for cleansing rheum (17.18).

17.25   Cancer of the Womb

Cancer may appear after a warm-natured swelling of the womb. The signs are hardness of the womb, heat, palpitation, and pain. The diaphragm is projected and the back of the feet swollen. In advanced stages, there is bleeding. Most women receive an annual check-up known as the Pap Test, which checks for presence of cancer cell growth. Information on drugless, natural therapies is available from local chapters of the International Association of Cancer Victors and Friends. Many herbs have been used in the treatment of cancer, not only of the womb but other parts of the body. The attitude of natural medicine is that cancer is the final degenerated condition of an organ or bodily system. As such, the establishment of a way of life based upon proper nutrition and harmony of the spirit is the best suggestion for avoiding such a final condition. Among the most prominent nontoxic therapies for cancer are the Gerson Therapy, Hoxsey Herbs, the Koch Therapy, and Laetrile. IACVF can supply details of how to discover physicians skilled in administering these therapies. When a bodily condition has degenerated into a full cancerous tumor, the therapy of choice is surgery. No curative claims are made for chemotherapy or radiation, these being palliative procedures designed to slow tumor growth.

While there are some cases of remission of tumors following various herbal and other natural treatments, there is no scientific evidence to support the recommendation of one herb to be used in any particular case. Since the liver has been damaged in all cases of cancer, care of this organ is vital to prevent cancer, as well as during its treatment. Cancer can be prevented, but seldom cured. (See also 20.15).

17.26 Strangulation of the Womb

This is similar to fainting and epilepsy; there is no foaming at the mouth and little nervous anxiety, but there is frequent fainting. The treatment is the same as for epilepsy and fainting (see 2.12 and 8.2).

The cause is sometimes attributed to pent-up sexual energy, so intercourse is recommended, if possible. Imprisonment of menses is another cause and was discussed in 17.1.

The Back, Legs, and Feet

General Considerations

The spine is made up of a series of bones called vertebrae. This vertebral column is the main axis of the body, providing general flexibility, yet also keeping the posture erect for walking. It is also the enclosing protective casing for the spinal cord and roots of the spinal nerves. It is the support to which the ribs, skull, and pelvis are connected to the spine, along with important plexus of nerves, muscles, and ligaments. The spinal column is composed of four sets of vertebrae, called the cervical (7 vertebrae), thoracic (12), lumbar (5), the sacrum (5 fused vertebrae), and the coccyx (3 to 5 rudimentary vertebrae).

Since the spinal cord and nerves are so closely connected with the spinal column, it is imperative that there be no misalignment of the column. A study done at the Palmer College of Chiropractic revealed that 60 millimeters of pressure (about enough to feel the finger touching the skin) applied to a spinal nerve will impede nearly 40 percent of nerve impulses across that vertebra. Since the nerve connections of the spinal column activate many functions in the body, it is easy to see that any misalignment of the spinal column can itself lead to lowered vitality and function of any organ.

Chiropractic, osteopathy, and naprapathy are branches of natural medicine specializing in treatment and alignment of the spine. Osteopaths are most like medical doctors, although they avoid use of drugs; chiropractors usually work only on the spine, though some today practice nutritional counseling, hydrotherapy, and other modalities. Naprapathy, a science developed in the early 1900s, involves gentle applications of pressure to the ligamentous tissue surrounding the spinal column to balance muscles that may be in spasm. In addition to these forms of treatment, all of which involve manipulation of the spine, there are many other systems of bodywork that center on the goal of insuring full nerve impulse flow along the spinal column. Shiatsu, kinesiology, Rolfing, acupressure, yoga, and t'ai chi are a few of these, but each has its special terminology and exercise patterns. It would be well to consider one or more of these forms of therapy if you have signs of pain, tension, and restricted movement in any muscles of the body.

18.1 Convexity

Convexity is the natural-medicine term used to describe the movement of one or more of the individual spinal processes out of place. This movement can be either upward, downward, to the right or left, or forward, or backward.

Convexity has several causes:

Fig. 13 • The Spinal Column

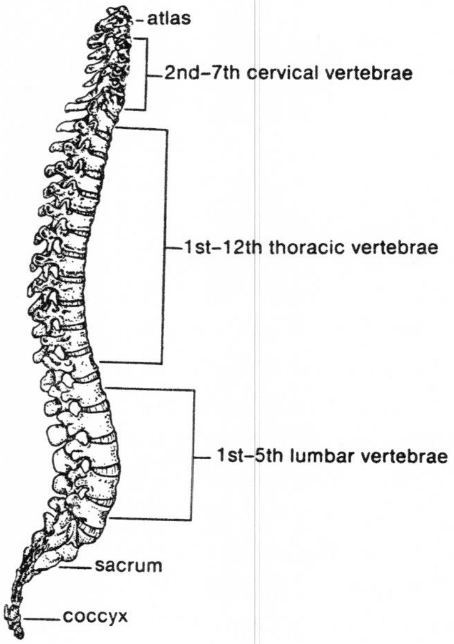

1. Swelling of the vertebra area (pain with fever).
2. Thick flatulency imprisoned under the vertebrae (severe pain without fever).
3. Spinous fluids absorbed by the ligaments in the back of the head (paleness of the face).
4. Convulsion or spasm of the ligament (can be felt, raised tissue).
5. Falls, injuries, or blows to the spine (signs are clear).

The natural remedies to be applied along with any form of massage or corrective manipulation are:

1. Swelling: laxatives, arnicated oil for pain. Consult section on swellings (Section 20).
2. Flatulence: Consult 10.7 and 14.6.
3. Moisture: remedy same as for 2.
4. Spasm: See sections on swellings (Section 20 and 2.24).
5. Injuries, falls: Correct the vertebra. If it has gone downward from its proper position, apply cupping on both sides to the top of the vertebra affected. If it has gone upward, place the cupping below on both sides. If it is forward or backward in projection, apply astringent salve. It would be best in any case of injury to the spine to have it treated by a specialist in spinal manipulation, as the muscles are interconnected among three vertebrae, not simply attached to one, and wrong application of a technique can easily aggravate the condition. Use arnicated oil for pain; it works almost immediately.

18.2 Backache

If the cause is bad temperament, the sign of coldness is pain without heaviness, and gas. The remedy is keeping warm, sun baths, and showers directing streams of hot water on the area affected. If the cause is production of phlegm, the sign is pain with heaviness; it often occurs after experiencing severe anger, fatigue, and the like, which stimulate formation of phlegm. The remedy is to purge the phlegm humour and use suppositories for phlegm. If the phlegm (ache) stays in one place, use salves to soothe it (arnicated oil, lobelia, peppermint oil, for instance). Also recommended is back massage with rose oil and saffron, and abstaining from intercourse. If this relief doesn't result, resort to purgatives.

Weakness of the kidneys can also cause backache, as was discussed in 14.3.

Excess blood in the veins of the back also causes ache, and the sign is that pain is felt along the entire spinal column, from the first vertebra to the last. The remedy is to apply cupping every five inches along both sides of the spinal column. For backache in women due to suppressed menstrual flow or excess superfluous matter, the remedy is to use diuretics to open the flow (see 17.1), and rub the back with rose oil.

18.3 Pelvis Ache

It sometimes occurs that the femur bone becomes slightly separated from the tissue that holds it in place in the pelvis, which is called a microevulsion of the femur head. It is probably best treated by a qualified practitioner, but you can try this remedy first: Lie down on a hard floor (carpeted is all right), and place a thick telephone book or other large book at an angle so the corner of the book is underneath and supporting the pelvis. This should be applied to one side at a time, and leave the book in place for about ten to twenty minutes. This will allow the tissue to repair itself while the femur head is properly positioned. If this problem recurs, you most likely need to do exercises to strengthen the pelvic muscles that support the femur and keep it positioned properly. Consult a practitioner.

18.4 Joint Ache

This can occur with or without swelling. If it originates in the joints of the hips it is called ischium; if it continues on down into the feet, it is called sciatica. If it affects the feet or toes it is called podogra. Many people lump all these pains together and call it arthritis or rheumatism of the joints.

If it comes over many months or even years, gradually worsening, it is caused by intemperament of the body, poor diet, excessive sugar consumption, and the buildup of toxic materials in the body.

If it is caused by bad temperament of the humours, it is recognized by moist swelling in the joints, but no pain. Salves recommended include: marshmallow and violet oil or fennel seed and melilot. Valerian root, hops, and camomile are combined as a tea for pain.

If the cause is black bile mixing with the blood humour, the sign is extreme burning pain. Use laxatives to move the bowels, detoxify, and purge the black bile humour. Salves in this case are not of use except to palliate the pain; lobelia and valerian root are recommended.

If the imbalance of the phlegm humour is causing joint ache, the remedy is to cleanse the entire system of phlegm with the tincture-of-lobelia emetic. Afterward, use hot-natured diuretics.

If the cause is prevalence of black bile alone, the signs are change of skin color, little pain, need to stretch all the time, excess of hard swelling in the joints. Use the black bile purgatives.

NOTE: Joint ache is caused by different substances in wrong concentrations. The single most useful herb for joint ache is saffron. However, it should be taken with cumin and ginger (one part saffron to five parts each of cumin and ginger), to avoid harming the stomach balance.

When you do take saffron, rub the joints with oil to which some beeswax has been added. There are several pain-relieving preparations:

3 drams ground dry coriander with 3 drams turbinado sugar. Take it all.

or

One teaspoon each of valerian root and camomile and a half-teaspoon hops; make two cups of tea and drink as desired. Do not repeat this mixture for more than three days.

or

2 drams marshmallow seeds, 2 drams of sugar or honey. Take it all.

In sciatica, the points to apply massage to relieve pain are about eight fingers' distance above the ankle bone on the side affected, the base of the little finger on the side affected, and the area of the Achilles tendon on the foot.

18.5 Swelling of the Veins of the Leg

The remedy is purging the black bile humour, eating foods that open the bowels, and vomiting to cleanse the stomach. Afterward, apply the white of an egg over the vein to reduce swelling.

18.6 Heel Ache

The cause may be ulcers of the heel, which should be treated with salves of scabious (devil's bit). If the cause is from a fall or stepping down hard and bruising the heel, add rose water and apply cupping to the side and just above the heel. If the cause is heat intemperament, rub with rose oil and, in case of coldness, rub with oil of fennel. An ice pack will also reduce pain and swelling.

18.7 Sole Ache

If pain is in the soles and causes problems in walking, make a salve of lentils cooked in vinegar and apply, lukewarm, to the soles of the feet.

Hair and Nails

General Considerations

The bulb of the hair root consists of many cells massed together, which constantly multiply and grow. Hairs in different parts of the body have different periods of growth, after which they are shed and replaced. In human beings this process goes on continuously. The life of individual scalp hairs is two to five years, of eyebrows and eyelashes three to five months. As children grow, the hairs of the eyebrows, lashes, and scalp become progressively larger and coarser than the preceding set. The sex hormones affect the growth of hair in the armpits and pubic area at puberty in both sexes, and on the chest and face of males. Hair grows at an average rate of 1.5 to 3.0 millimeters per week.

19.1 Baldness (Alopecia)

Falling out of hair, with or without loss of adjacent skin, is called baldness. In both cases, there is some corruption of the skin. The cure is to be found in adjusting the phlegm humour. If there is no attendant skin eruption, shaving the entire head sometimes helps to promote new vigorous growth of hair. Rubbing the head with myrtle oil and date water is also recommended.

If only the hair on the crown of the head falls out, the remedy is the same as above. If it happens as part of the normal process of aging, there is no cure.

19.2   Split Ends of Hair

The remedy is to drink fresh fruit juices and apply jojoba oil or other oils to the hair, along with scalp massage twice a day.

19.3   Oily Head

The remedy is purging the body. See beginning of Formulary.

19.4   Whiteness of Hair

Hair will turn white as part of the aging process, which is normal. For hair that turns white prematurely, the *hakims* recommend this procedure: eat date jam every morning for a month; during the last week of the month, drink water that has been gathered at a holy shrine. Then, allow one month to pass, avoiding all sour foods and sexual intercourse. Finally, take a phlegm purgative and detoxify the system.

19.5   Care of the Hair

Here are recommendations for various general applications for the hair on the head and body:

To prevent hair loss   Rub with oil of mastic or oil of myrtle.

To make the hair grow long   Wash the head with myrtle and date water; if available, geranium blossoms can be added.

To stimulate the roots of the hair   Rub with olive oil and cucumber water. Adjust the phlegm humour.

To remove hair   Apply slaked lime and olive oil as a depilatory paste, but do not apply to the armpits, genitals, or other sensitive areas of the body. Ordinarily, use of a razor or plucking the hairs out as they first appear is the comfortable method.

To stop hair growth at the roots Rubbing with opium, vinegar, gallnut, or blood of turtle is recommended by the *hakims*.

To soften the hair Apply a decoction of yellow-wood herb several times a day for a week.

To straighten the hair Mix olive oil with lukewarm water and rub on the hair.

To blacken the hair Grind litharge, slaked lime, and clay in equal parts and make into a thick paste with water. Apply to hair for ten minutes, then wash well to remove all of the paste. Then put leaves of castor plant on the head for three hours. Wash with warm water and rub with any nonflower oil.

To redden hair A color between red and yellow is obtained by washing the hair with sedge and white hellebore. Henna works as well.

19.6 *Whitening of Nails*

The remedy is to pound linseed and milk, mix with honey, and apply to the nails. If this does not work, use a purgative and detoxify the system.

19.7 *Nails Turning Yellow*

The remedy is to reduce biliousness and apply watercress and vinegar, in equal parts, to the nails.

19.8 *Aching Nails*

Pound leaves of myrtle with leaves of cedar and make a salve of the resultant juices; apply to nails.

19.9 *Thickening of Nails*

This mostly happens at the base, or roots, of the nails. The remedy is to purge the black bile humour.

19.10   Cracking of Nails

This occurs along the vertical axis of the nails; the remedy is to give moistening foods and purge the black bile humour.

19.11   Lack of Nail Growth

If there is no pain in the nail, the remedy is in purging the phlegm humour. If it is accompanied by pain, pricking the fingertip of the affected fingers to let a little blood out is suggested. If it is a toenail that is lacking growth, the remedy is to apply syrup of jujube.

19.12   Itching of the Nails

Wash in fresh, flowing stream or river water, and apply a salve of pounded figs. Scrupulous hygiene is important.

19.13   Bruised Nails

The remedy is applying a salve made of pounded pomegranate leaves and myrtle leaves as soon as the injury occurs. After a few hours, apply a poultice of whole-wheat flour and olive oil.

19.14   Breaking Nails (and Whiteness)

The remedy is to mix rose preserve and oxymel with almond oil (in equal parts), and apply to nails.

19.15   Blood under the Nail

After a forceful blow to the nail, blood will usually settle and become "dead" under the nail. Mix equal parts of resin and wheat flour and rub the nail with it. Wash the nail frequently in a solution of watercress and vinegar. The object is to soften the dead nail, so even sucking on the affected finger is helpful. If you want the nail to come off, make a salve of milk and ground apricot kernels; apply and wrap with a clean cloth.

Section 20

Boils, Swellings, Infections, and Aches

General Considerations

When there are toxic matters in the body, including bacteria and other pathogens, the body tries to expel them as quickly as possible. However, the normal systems of elimination, especially the lymphatic channels and ducts, are sometimes already congested. The body then tries to send the toxins out through other openings, including the pores of the skin. Since the skin is not designed to eliminate this type of matter, the pores themselves become clogged, and a boil is formed.

A single bubblelike eruption is called a boil. When this small swelling is accompanied by heat, pain, and redness, apply a salve of such herbs as sandalwood, false acacia, rose, and common field scabious. If the boil has not begun to dry up after one day, apply a second pomade or poultice made of barley flour, fresh coriander, and marshmallow (in equal parts). The boil may be reduced by being "drained" away internally. If it needs to be ripened, do so with ground fig seeds and linseed made into a salve or poultice. If it ripens within a day or two by itself, it will "point" and drain away from the surface. Do not squeeze or pinch it. If it becomes larger or spreads, it will probably have to be lanced by a physician.

The above applies to boils and swellings on the body, *except when located behind the ear, under the arms, or on the groin.* For these cases, see 20.9.

20.1 Gangrene

Gangrene is the end result of an unchecked infection and ultimately leads to the putrefaction of the limb or body part. It is very serious and can lead to death. The signs of systemic infection are high fever, loss of appetite, diarrhea, and flushing. When this condition of any infection of the entire system is present, a physician is urgently needed. If medical help is inaccessible, use antibiotics if available, to check the spreading of infection. When the limb has turned black, however, it must be amputated to prevent infection of other parts of the body.

20.2 Swelling with Redness

Redness occurring as the sole sign is indicative of bilious swelling. If only the yellow bile humour is affected, it is called "pure redness": the skin appears shiny and is a little yellowish in color, and there is a burning sensation. For this, purge the yellow bile humour and consume cold and moist foods and herbs.

If there is yellow bile mixed with the blood humour, there is no burning sensation, but the swollen part is very red. In this case as well, purge the yellow bile humour.

20.3 Skin Cancer

If there is any swelling, reddened area, growth or wound on the skin that does not heal, a physician should be consulted to test for cancer (see also 20.15). Skin cancer has many forms and names in allopathic medicine. In general, a mild skin cancer is treatable by surgical excision of the affected area, if discovered soon enough. The signs are often that the skin is greatly swollen, there is redness that spreads quickly, and the heat of the swelling may feel as though a fire had been touched to the skin. Some cancers of the skin are painless, however. The herbal application is first to purge the black bile humour and detoxify the system (this all must be carried out under medical supervision). The preparation to put on the cancer is a half-pint of vinegar heated to boiling temperature, mixed with 2 drams of camphor, and, after cooling, applied to the skin.

Another skin cancer salve (also reputed to be effective for removing plantar warts) is made as follows:

Take one ounce of red clover blossoms and simmer in two pints of distilled water for one hour. Strain, add another ounce of red clover blossoms to the liquid, and slowly boil another hour. Strain again, and simmer until the liquid is driven off. When the liquid is nearly all evaporated, you must watch the mixture carefully to avoid scorching it. When it has reached the consistency of tar, remove from the flame and put in a clean, low, wide-mouthed jar. It will harden somewhat as it cools. Apply to the affected part and cover with a piece of moleskin or soft, sterile cloth.

20.4 Small Boils with White Heads and Red Roots

Purge both the phlegm and bile humours. Soak pomegranate skin in vinegar and rose water and apply to the boils.

20.5 Moist Boil with Severe Burning and Itching

When it appears, the roots dry soon. Red, featherlike lines are seen before it appears. This may be a prelude to skin cancer. Purge the yellow bile humour and apply a salve of rose water and vinegar.

20.6 Large Boils

These boils sometimes contain a thin watery discharge or thinned blood. The remedy is to thicken the blood and apply cold salves, such as camphor, cucumber, and the like. The boil may be pierced with a sterile needle if it comes to a head.

20.7 Random Boils

They look red; some are big and some small. The main sign is that they appear very suddenly and itch. They are caused by blood and phlegm humour imbalance. In the case of blood humour imbalance, soften the stomach and apply a salve made with rose leaves. In case of phlegm, use a phlegm purgative, and stop eating phlegm-producing foods.

20.8 Canker

This is a swelling caused by biliousness and blood humour imbalance. It appears in the head. The entire face becomes very red and swollen. The stomach must be kept soft and the humours corrected. Use laxatives first, and apply cold salves on the throat and chest to keep the swelling from coming down from the face to the chest. Mix 30 drams of jujube with oxymel and drink the mixture.

20.9 Boils and Carbuncles of the Armpit, behind the Ear, and in the Groin

If it is caused by an ulcer, consult the appropriate sections for these parts. If it is not due to an ulcer, make a salve of violet leaves, violet oil, and beeswax. Do not use cold pomades. When the substance has been drawn to a ripened point, it can be pierced and drained. These are often signs of a systemic infection and should be seen by a physician.

20.10 Abscesses

Infected swellings need treatment by a physician. The natural treatment is to purge the blood and phlegm humours and drink oxymel. For three days apply a poultice of purslane leaves, sandalwood, and betel nut (in equal parts). On the fourth day, apply a half-ounce of yellow dock with white of egg as binder. When it shrinks and ripens to a point, pierce it with a sterile needle. After it is cleaned of rheum and pus, apply a mixture of pounded figs and resin gum. This can be alternated once a day with dough made of whole-wheat flour and water, with a little salt, linseed oil, and honey added.

20.11 Soft, White Swelling without Heat and Pain

Purge the phlegm humour and correct for cold intemperament. Apply a salve of aloe vera, vinegar, and rose water.

20.12 Swelling that Is Thick and Hard and Moves under the Skin

When palpated, this kind of swelling is given several names by the *hakims*, according to the consistencies: honeylike, fatlike, flourlike, oil-like, and curdlike. The remedy is to purge the phlegm humour.

20.13 Skin Tumors

The difference between a tumor and the condition mentioned in 20.12 is that a skin tumor is a hard growth on the surface of the skin. Any tumor should be diagnosed by a physician. After such diagnosis is made, a decision can be reached whether to pursue an orthodox or nontoxic treatment (see 20.15).

20.14 Scrofula

This condition is characterized by chronic swelling of the glands, especially lymphatics. The imbalance is caused either by phlegm or by phlegm mixed with black bile. In both cases, the phlegm humour must be purged. A definitive diagnosis should be sought whenever there is chronic swelling of the lymph glands.

20.15 Cancer

See also Sections 10, General Considerations, 17.25, and 20.3. Cancer—in all of its many forms—has become one of the worst plagues in recorded history. Theories about its origin and methods of treatment abound, but it remains a fact that the cure for cancer has still eluded humankind. Some forms are apparently "cured" by surgical removal, although in many cases the cancer reappears, sometimes many years later. The medical doctors who operate the largest clinic in the Western Hemisphere offering nontoxic treatment of cancer have only approximately a 3.5 percent rate of total remission after five years. The "cure" rate in conventional forms of treatment is approximately the same.

It seems futile to focus treatment on the final stages of a process that takes many years to develop. At the time a cancer is diagnosed, there is always to be found degeneration of primary organs, and the organ most frequently affected is the liver.

According to the view of natural medicine, cancer occurs as the degeneration of the human body or its parts over a period of many years, due to faulty and unbalanced living habits. If you will review the chapters on the origin and progression of illness, you will see that the incomplete digestion of nutrients causes congestion of one or more organs (or humours). Since the body is capable of healing and balancing itself and is astoundingly competent at reducing and correcting the effects of abusive dietary habits, the congestion of an organ may be corrected in whole or part for some time, often for years. But the quality of functioning of those organs also degenerates over time, so the self-healing process weakens. The fact that cancer appears in so many forms and affects so many different organs has its explanation in each person's inherited strengths and weaknesses in his or her own body.

The liver is the seat of manufacture of the blood, and it is simple to see that any chronic or degenerated condition of that organ will lead to impurity and faulty production of the blood, which is the medium for carrying the life force by the breath.

Most cancerous tumors appear as a very hard swelling, with a dark color and rounded shape. The surface is puffy or sunken, and the area may exhibit reddish and greenish veins that resemble a crab (*cancer* is the Latin word for crab.) The black bile humour must be purged constantly, and the liver must be strengthened. In my opinion, anyone who has received a definitive diagnosis of cancer should investigate all available forms of therapy: surgery, chemotherapy, radiation, and all forms of nontoxic therapies. Some of the better-known unorthodox therapies are Koch Glyoxylide Therapy, Gerson Therapy, Laetrile (Amygdalen), Iscadore, Tekarina, Crofton Vaccine, Saline–Hydrogen Peroxide Therapy, Parabenzoquinine (PBQ), the Nicolini Method, the Baumann Electrolyte Rejuvenation Program, Blass Oxygen Therapy, Neihans Cellular Therapy, and the Hoxsey Herbs.

Many of these treatments were developed by the person whose name they bear, after these people cured themselves of cancer. There are many other such forms, and to investigate them all would require much labor. As unfortunate as it is, there do exist some perverted people who play upon the suffering of others and offer absurd hopes for high fees in promising a cure for cancer. Remember that for any known treatment, orthodox or unorthodox, the absolute cure rate is abysmally low.

Information about unorthodox cancer therapies is available from The International Association of Cancer Victors and Friends, 7740 West Manchester Avenue, Suite 110, Playa Del Rey, California, 90291. They have chapters in most cities, and usually have a listing in the telephone book.

The clinic of Dr. Hans Nieper at 21 Sedanstrasse 3000, Hanover, Germany, has the reputation for being the finest facility for treatment of cancer in the world, offering a combination of both orthodox and nontoxic therapies, which are prescribed by medical doctors on an individual basis.

In the Western Hemisphere, a clinic similar in approach to the one in Germany is operated by Dr. Marco Brown, Director, Fairfield Medical Center, P.O. Box 1296, Montego Bay, Jamaica, W.I.

Cancer will be eliminated only when people return to a more balanced, natural lifestyle, and keep the body, mind, and spirit free from impurities.

20.16 Scabs

These appear often with itching after boils come to a point and drain. Some are dry and some moist. If the scab is dry, rub beet juice and pea water on it. Wash with warm water afterward and use a purgative. Massage the area of the scab with rose oil and vinegar. For wet scabs, cup the area around the scab, then give a laxative for the phlegm humour. Do not use hot salves or pomades on scabs.

20.17 Itching

If itching persists without any other sign, boil a quarter-ounce of linseed in two ounces of honey, add some powdered purslane, and apply as a pomade.

For scabs and itching in children, give a tub bath with rose leaves and violet leaves added, and afterward rub the affected parts with olive oil.

20.18 Severe Itching with Prickling and Small Red Boils

The remedy is to apply the biliousness laxative and apply a salve of salt, henna, and vinegar.

20.19 Itching with Severe Pain

If the itching has just commenced, rub the area with balsam, dates, and vinegar salve (in equal parts). If the itching persists and the skin becomes thickened from scratching, use a black bile humour laxative and take warm baths. The recommended salve is made from such things as mustard, alum, and myrrh mixed with a little wheat-germ oil and vinegar.

20.20 Pimples

These are white pustules that appear most frequently on the nose and forehead. Purge the phlegm humour and apply a salve of sarsaparilla and vinegar.

20.21 Pimples on the Buttocks, Anus, or Vulva

Use a general purgative and detoxify the system.

20.22 Broken Blood Vessels

Rupture of the veins just under the skin is caused either by a blow or may appear spontaneously. The skin is discolored by the accumulation of blood and vaporous substances. When the veins contract, swelling may appear; when veins expand, the swelling goes down. If the swelling is chronic, the skin may take on a purplish color. The suggested treatment is to apply salves of astringent herbs, such as gallnut or chestnut. Avoid blood stimulants.

20.23 Sebaceous Cysts

These appear in different forms. One is small, white, and hard, with roots; a little rheum comes out from time to time. These can appear anywhere. Another appears mostly on the face, is quite hard, red in color, and often as large as a quarter. A third variety usually appears behind the ear and will emit a puslike substance, sometimes with blood mixed in. These can also appear on the back of the neck, and sometimes are quite painful. The treatment for all types of these sebaceous cysts is to use a purgative and cleanse the system. For the last kind, use a purgative as well, but also drop a little violet oil and mother's milk into the nose and rub the same mixture on the neck and head.

Miscellaneous

21.1 *Blackheads*

These appear mostly on the face, but can appear anywhere there is an accumulation of dirt and lack of skin hygiene. Wash the skin daily and apply a salve of rhubarb and honey. If black heads keep appearing, detoxify the body.

21.2 *Bloodblisters*

These occur from a blow to the skin or from a sharp pinching of the skin. Apply pounded beet leaves and pennyroyal herb made into a salve.

21.3 *Freckles*

This change in skin pigmentation frequently occurs after exposure to the sun. It is sometimes hereditary. Apply the remedy for blackheads if one wishes to get rid of them. There is no harm in freckles.

21.4 *Tattoos*

The method said to remove a tattoo via herbal preparation is as follows: using a little warm water as a base, take some ground unroasted coffee beans and rub the area of the tattoo for a few minutes. Then cover with a pomade made of turpentine gum ($\frac{1}{4}$ ounce) with honey (2 ounces) for three days. Remove and wash with warm salt water. If necessary, reapply the pomade until the tattoo is eradicated. The effect of the turpentine is to create an ulcer of the surface that then sloughs off the impregnated tissue as it heals. Afterward, an application of golden seal will help prevent infection. This remedy should only be carried out under the supervision of a physician, as it may become infected. There are also skin-grafting procedures and other medical modes of tattoo removal.

21.5 Frostbite

In its mild form, this appears as a dark redness on the face and hands after exposure to subzero temperatures. Numbness of the affected part is a sign, and pain follows. The remedy is to give cooked dates until diarrhea occurs, and apply a salve of red clover blossoms with a little Castile soap added. When the redness subsides, wash frequently with warm water.

21.6 Blackness of Skin after Exposure to Cold

This needs first aid treatment at a medical facility. If none is available, rub olive oil on the hands before any swelling begins and before they turn blue. When the swelling appears, place hands in a solution of cooked dill and melilot or a decoction of linseed. Cabbage water also works. When the hands are taken out of the water (when the swelling is checked), rub with rose oil. A pomade of pounded boiled lentils applied to the affected part is recommended.

21.7 Swelling and Itching of Fingers during Cold Weather

The remedy is to wash them with salty water and also with the water from turnips and beets.

21.8 Dandruff

The remedy is to put a teaspoon of salt in beet water and wash the head with it. If it is chronic, purge the phlegm and black bile humours.

21.9 Cracks of Hands, Face, and Lips

If the cause is external factors such as cold and wind exposure, use an ointment of sweet almond oil. If due to internal causes, use a purgative and consume more fruits.

21.10 Rough Skin

Use a purgative and massage the body with rose oil.

21.11 Scratches

For minor surface scratches, apply almond or rose oil with a pinch of ground golden seal.

21.12 Lice

The first recommendation is to purge the body, wash with salt water, and change the clothes frequently. One kind of louse imbeds itself in the roots of the hair and moves about when stimulated by heat. Cayenne pepper in vinegar will dislodge these lice, which can then be washed away.

21.13 Severe Perspiration

Often the cause is that the body is full of phlegm; if so, the phlegm purgative should be employed. This condition can also be caused by overeating and engorging the stomach. The remedy is to refrain from eating for a twenty-four-hour period or longer. If perspiration is caused by general debilitation and weakness, undertake to strengthen the health of the person, and burn dried leaves of myrtle and allow the smoke to reach the person's body. Caloric foods imprison perspiration, a normal avenue of excretion of superfluities. However, people sometimes faint from dehydration as a result of excessive perspiration. The following remedy helps to slow down the elimination of perspiration and in preventing fainting: Pour two ounces each of apple juice and rose water into two ounces of sesame oil; heat gradually to a slow boil, and continue boiling until the water is driven off and only the oil remains. Take a teaspoonful as needed.

NOTE: The prevalence of perspiration that is part of the natural repulsion of toxins associated with a healing crisis should not be stopped.

21.14   Bloody Perspiration

This is excretion of blood with perspiration. The remedy is to use strong laxatives, correct for hot intemperament of the blood, and remove any obstruction of the pores of the skin by using astringents.

21.15   Obesity and Thinness

When carried to extremes, these conditions are an imbalance that affects the overall health. To gain weight, use this preparation: almonds, pine nuts (and any other oil-producing seeds or nuts) in equal parts, pounded together. Mix with cow's butter and turbinado sugar and take a portion morning and evening before meals. Eat moist, energetic foods.

To reduce obesity, reduce food intake. The best diet of all is to eat only when there is true hunger, and then only enough to take the edge off the hunger. Rub the body with oils and common dill ground fine. Make the person sleep on the hard ground. A detoxification program adhered to strictly, and employing chickory-root or coffee enemas, generally causes from five to fifteen pounds of weight loss in a ten-day period. Establishing a day of fasting once a week (or even for half-days at first) will help bring a compulsive eater under the control of self-discipline.

21.16   Bad Odor of the Body

Bathe frequently and rub the body with rose oil after bathing. Use a purgative as well. A little powdered bicarbonate of soda dusted under the arms will absorb most of the foul odor of the armpits. Any extended period of corrupted body odor calls for corrective treatment by detoxification and looking into the underlying humoral imbalances.

21.17 Burning by Fire

Two treatments are suggested. The first to put fresh aloe vera on the skin that has been exposed to fire. Anything other than minor burns should be treated by a physician, as burns can become infected easily. The second suggestion is to apply fresh purslane that has been cooled in a freezer or on ice to the area, changing often enough to keep cool. If a blister appears, rub some fireplace soot with egg white on it.

21.18 Burning by Hot Oil

The remedy is the same as for fire; also, you may put on egg white mixed with a little olive oil as a first aid measure.

21.19 Burning by Lightning

Anyone struck by lightning needs medical treatment at once. Emergency measures for burns are the same as mentioned for burns by fire.

21.20 Sunburn

For mild overexposure to the sun, apply fresh aloe vera. Use protective oils before going out into the sun, or cover the exposed skin with appropriate clothing.

21.21 Tongue Burns by Caustics

The people in India chew a leafy substance called *pan* with gallnut and limestone added. While the betel leaf and other ingredients do contain all the vitamins necessary for humans, it also can cause tongue burns if made too strong. Some of the substances chewed in the mouth in America (such as cocoa leaf with lime) may also cause a slight burn, especially to those who try it for the first time. Recommended is to rub oil of sweet almond and a little finely ground nutmeg on the tongue.

21.22 Wounds

The treatment of most wounds is in the province of the medical physician or surgeon, who has the training and materials to set bones, sew the skin, and perform more complicated procedures to repair internal damage to the body. These forms of treatment lie outside the realm of simple treatment by herbs.

In general, the most dangerous wounds are those to the head and brain, or to the heart. Serious wounds to either place are often fatal. If a penlight held to the eyes of a person struck in the head does not cause contraction of the pupil, it is usually a sign that brain damage has occurred. Obviously, emergency medical aid should be sought as soon as possible in such cases.

The kidney, urinary bladder, and intestine are next in order of importance in wounds. Wounds to the kidney and bladder are known from the urine; wounds to the intestine are diagnosed by the feces. Wounds involving nerves are known by pale color in the face, fainting, and convulsions. Knee wounds easily become chronic and are difficult to cure without surgery. Internal injuries to the abdomen are signaled by vomiting and hiccups. Wounds to the chest produce expulsion of large amounts of air and asthma signs. Apply the best first aid you can, and seek a person equipped to handle emergency wounds.

21.23 Falls and Blows from the Fist

If there is no swelling or fever, make a salve of spirits of ammonia and egg white. If there is swelling and fever, apply cupping and reinforce the specific area of injury (also see Sections 20, General Considerations, and 20.2). For deep muscle bruises, apply arnicated oil for pain and give marijuana tea as a relaxant.

21.24 Welt from Beating with a Whip

If serious, the tissue under the skin is spread out. If any flesh
is torn loose, replace it over the exposed flesh. If no emergency
medical aid is available, the procedure recommended by the
hakims is to apply fresh meat. This is said to have effect within
twenty-four hours. If blood accumulates under the welts, put
a salve of ground radish seeds on the wound.

21.25 Broken Bones

The complete dislocation or fracture of a bone, with or without
puncture of the flesh, or bruising of the bone or muscles
around it, should be treated by a competent physician or
bonesetter. Until one is available, rub olive oil on the part, and
also put on pounded leaves of myrtle and marshmallow with
egg yolk and cover with a sterile cloth.

21.26 Poisons

If an unknown substance of any quantity is ingested, call the
emergency room of any hospital and give them whatever
information you can about the bottle it was kept in or what the
source of the substance was. They will advise you as to what
can be done immediately and arrange for an ambulance, if
needed. It is a good idea to get a poison chart and tack it up
on the wall.

Poisons can be animal, vegetable, or mineral. When someone
has eaten a poison, if it is not known what the source is,
vomiting should first be employed to attempt to expel the
substance as quickly as possible. There are some exceptions to
this rule, such as if the poison is an acid caustic, and it is hard
to act with certainty if the identity of the ingested substance is
not known at all. Lots of sesame oil or butter added to warm
water will usually provoke vomiting. Lobelia tincture should
not be used, as this will also speed digestion of the substance.
If the person cannot vomit much, drinking common dill with
salt and oil mixed in water will usually procure vomiting. Give
as much fresh milk as possible; this provides mucus to coat the

stomach and slows absorption of toxins. If the person becomes drowsy and seems to be falling asleep, try to prevent this by giving strong stimulants such as coffee or spearmint in strong decoction. If the person has an irrepressible urge for a particular food, it is probably what the body needs to counteract the poison.

NOTE: If the person faints, the eyes roll back into the sockets or become red, the pulse is not beating, cold perspiration appears, and the tongue is thrown out from the mouth, there is usually little hope for survival.

21.27 Stings of Poisonous Insects and Snakes

These are treated in the following ways:

1. Give something to increase the natural temperature, to reinforce the intestines and kill the poison, or slow down its absorption into the blood stream. Opium is said to have this effect. Milk, as a drink and enema, will coat the membranes and help slow down absorption.

2. Purge the body of moisture by inducing vomiting or diarrhea.

3. Give antitoxin or antidote if known and available.

4. Give a medicine to stir up the phlegm and repulse the nature of the poison (four drops of tincture of iodine will accomplish this).

5. Do something to stop the spread of the poison, such as opening the vein and sucking out the toxic blood. A small incision can be made over the point of the bite, and a tourniquet can be applied about five to ten inches above the wound. Cupping can be done over the cut, or the poison can be sucked out with the mouth, although care should be taken not to ingest any of the blood by lubricating the mouth with rose or other flower oil before sucking.

Eating three palmfuls of fresh coriander is said to be good for the sting of wasps, bees, and ants. If you have any sulphur-tipped kitchen matches handy, wet the tip of one with saliva and rub on the area of the sting; if done within thirty seconds or so of the sting, there is little swelling or pain.

Despite their reputation, the bites or stings of tarantulas, scorpions, and black widow spiders are not often fatal to adults (they *may* be to children); there is often more danger from the shock experienced after any insect or animal bite than from the wound or poison itself.

21.28   Wound by Bite of Rabid Animal

There are rabies antitoxins, which must be administered by a physician. The people in remote areas without access to medical treatment (such as Afghanistan) take some blood from the dog or animal that bit the person and mix it with water and drink it as an emergency antitoxin. At other times, the animal is killed and its liver fried and eaten. If treated in this way, the wounds usually do not heal for a long time.

Rabies vaccine is effective, even if given some days after the bite—usually within ten days. Skunks and bats are prime carriers of rabies, and cats and dogs have plagues of rabies among their population from time to time, especially in the Western states. Rabies is almost invariably fatal if not treated with an antitoxin.

Iridology, The Science of Iris Diagnosis

The science of iridology had its beginnings in the middle of the nineteenth century in Budapest, Hungary. In the 1820s, Ignatz von Peckzely of Budapest was a small boy fascinated with birds. By chance, one day he caught an owl, and in the struggle to subdue it, the owl's right leg was broken. As Peckzely later recalled, he noticed on looking into the owl's wide eyes after the injury to the limb that a small black spot had formed in the otherwise clear eye.

He prepared a splint and repaired the leg, and kept the bird for a pet. During the healing of the leg, Peckzely noticed that the black spot in the eye became overcoated with a white film and surrounded by a white border. He later realized that this denoted formation of scar tissue.

Peckzely was later imprisoned in 1848 for revolutionary activities; this gave him ample time to pursue his hobby of examining eyes and to develop his theory that injuries leave visible signs in the eyes. He became more and more certain about the discovery with the owl in his childhood. When he was released from prison, he gained a post as an intern in the surgical wards of a college hospital, where he had an opportunity to observe many thousands of patients before and after accidents and operations, and it was from viewing these changes that he finally was able to prepare a chart of the eyes. In 1866, he began practicing medicine in Budapest and published his first book on the iris, *Discovery in the Realm of Nature and Art of Healing*. At about the same time, the Swedish homeopath Nils Liljequist made practically identical discoveries about the iris and brought the work to America.

In the United States and Great Britain, others have since further developed and expanded Peckzely's pioneering work. Among the physicians who have contributed to the science of iridology are Lindlahr, Dritzer, Boyd, Brown-Neil, Lahn, Francis, and Jensen.

Theory of Iridology

Every organ and part of the body is represented in the iris in a well-defined area. The nerve filaments, muscle fibers, and minute blood vessels in these areas of the iris react to changing conditions in the corresponding organs with visible signs such as spots, lines, lesions, and changes in pigment density. By means of these various marks, signs, and discolorations in the iris, nature reveals inherited weakness and tendency to ailments such as diabetes, tuberculosis, and so forth. Nature also reveals by such means acute or chronic catarrhal conditions, destruction of tissue, drug poisonings, broken bones, and surgical operations. From the eye, according to the science of iridology, one can read the inherited and acquired tendencies toward health and disease, the general body condition, and the state of every organ in the body. Signs of prolonged emotion and stress are also recorded. Futhermore, one skilled in iris diagnosis can predict the healing crises through which the body must pass on its way to health.

Diagnosis from the eye confirms Hahnemann's teaching that all acute diseases have a constitutional background of hereditary deficiencies. Finally, it reveals the gradual purification of the system of morbid matter and readjustment to normal conditions.

The diagram shows where all the vital organs and parts of the body are represented in various parts of the iris.

Body Conditions Shown in the Iris

Any irritation in the body is transmitted through nerves, which stimulate a rush of blood, causing swelling and congestion. This is transmitted through reflex nerve stimulation to the corresponding area in the iris.

For diagnostic purposes, the umbilicus is the center of the body. This corresponds to the black pupil in the center of the iris. The chart shows the stomach as corresponding to the first circle surrounding the pupil. If dark lines or spots appear in this ring, it denotes gastric trouble. All medicines that show themselves in the iris are poisonous to the body.

The different colors representing certain drugs (such as red for iodine or greenish-yellow for quinine) found in the iris are created by pigments deposited in the surface layers of the iris.

In a similar manner, areas are marked on the chart to show the intestinal tract, pancreas, sympathetic nervous system, reproductive and urinary organs, and so forth.

Irises record three stages in the development of disease: acute, chronic, and destructive. The acute stage is the inflammatory condition, characterized by redness, soreness, heat, and pain. The chronic stage is always called the stage of failure. Nature brings the acute stage gradually, and it is shown in the iris by grayish-white lines in the iris. If drugs are used to check the acute stage, dark lines appear.

In the first stage, tendencies are shown by color, density, and hereditary lesion. The color indicates whether the tissues are normal or affected by disease. The density is the grain or structure composing the iris and gives information about the tone and vitality of the body. Hereditary lesions show as dull gray and indicate corresponding weaknesses in the same organs in the parent's body, unless they are due to recessive genes.

The chronic stage, with lowered vitality and pathogenic organisms in the system, gradually causes destruction of tissue. Similar changes take place in the areas of the iris; in these areas, the tissues dry, shrivel, and turn black. When this happens, the white signs of the acute stage are intermingled with black streaks. In the advanced stage of destruction, the corresponding layers of the iris will be destroyed and leave a black spot.

In a newborn Caucasian child, the iris is nearly always blue. This is because pigmentation develops after birth, and so the color of the eyes may alter. Colors vary in many types of people, but in Caucasians there are only two true iris pigments: light azure blue and light hazel brown. Non-Caucasian's are dark

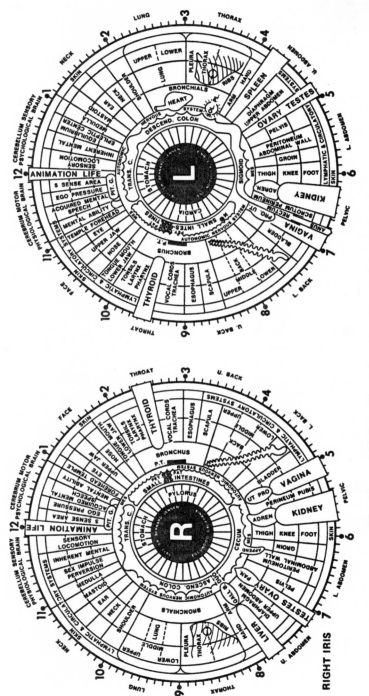

Fig. 14 • Iridology Chart developed by Dr. Bernard Jensen

brown or black. Other colors are really shades of these pigments. Color changes often occur in the iris, and these reflect the changing conditions of the person's health. Color spots indicate accumulations of drugs, taken either internally or externally. This shows that drugs are not always eliminated from the body, and because of the constant irritation can be factors in disease.

The Practice of Iridology

The practitioner of the science of iridology will use several terms that indicate symptoms: the *sympathetic wreath* shows the condition of the gastrointestinal tract; *nerve rings* indicate an overstimulation of the nervous system; white flakes in the outer rim of the iris are called a *lymphatic rosary* and show inflammation of the lymph vessels; and a *scurf rim* on the outermost rim of the iris shows poor condition of the skin.

Generally speaking, the examiner will seat the patient in a comfortable chair and use an eye light with a small magnifying glass. He surveys the iris for color, overacidity, scurf rim, nerve rings, drug signs, acute signs, chronic signs, destructive signs, sympathetic wreath, and other factors. In some clinics, 35-mm slides are taken of the iris and then projected onto a large screen, and the signs found are explained to the patient.

It takes considerable instruction and practice to become proficient at reading the iris. More information can be obtained from: Iridologists International, Route 1, Box 52, Escondido, California 92025.

Recommended Reading

Jensen, Bernard. *The Science and Practice of Iridology.* Escondido, Calif.: Bernard Jensen, 1974.
Wilborn, Robert, and James and Marcia Terrell. *Handbook of Iris Diagnosis and Rational Therapy.* Mokelumne Hill, Calif.: Health Research, 1961.

Appendix II

Reflexology
(Foot-Zone Therapy)

This is a part of the ancient Chinese system of acupressure. The soles of the feet are known to reflect a great sensitivity, and are felt by Eastern practitioners to be part of a mechanism of drawing in and discharging energy and magnetic charges from the earth.

The specific areas of the soles of the feet (see chart) are shown to relate to individual organ function. The technique is to apply a deep massage with the tips of the thumbs. Small nodes can be felt in those areas of the sole in which nerve flow is reduced, which in turn is a reflection of lack of vital energy in another part of the body.

This form of manipulation of the feet can be done by anyone, although there are persons who specialize in foot reflexology. The diagnostic use of reflexology by physicians includes noting any areas where there is extreme pain on firmly pressing, and the corresponding area of the body is investigated for possible chronic disease.

Specialists claim many conditions are helped by reflexology, such as stomach troubles, sexual problems, and appendicitis; but they do not claim responsibility for curing a disease, as it is up to the body itself, which is stimulated to engage its self-healing mechanisms.

Recommended Reading

Bryant, Ina. *Foot Massage and Nerve Tension.* Kingsport, Tenn.: Kingsport Press, 1978.

Carter, Mildred. *Helping Yourself with Foot Reflexology.* Englewood Cliffs, N.J.: Prentice-Hall, 1975.

Ingham, Eunice. *Stories the Feet Can Tell.* Rochester, N.Y.: Ingham Publisher, Box 948, Rochester, N.Y. 14603.

Fig. 15 • Reflexology Chart

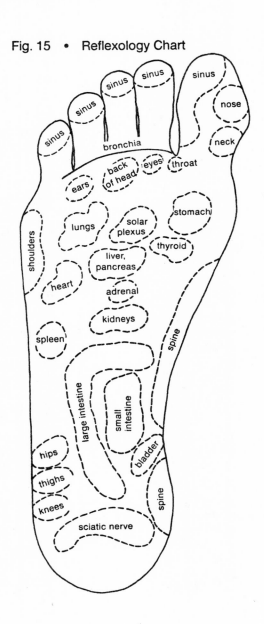

Bibliography

Children and Natural Childbirth

Benson, Ralph C. *Handbook of Obstetrics and Gynecology*. Los Altos, Calif.: Lange Medical Publications, 1974.

Eiger, Marvin, and Sally Olds. *The Complete Book of Breastfeeding*. New York: Bantam Books, 1972.

Elolesser, Leo, Edith Galt, and Isabel Hemingway. *Pregnancy, Childbirth and the Newborn: A Manual for Rural Midwives*. Niños Heroes, Mexico: Inter-American Indian Institute, 1973.

Khan, Hazrat Inayat. *The Sufi Message of Hazrat Inayat Khan*, Vol. III. London: Barrie & Jenkins, 1971.

Myles, Margaret. *Textbook for Midwives*. New York: Longmans, 1974.

Ostrander, Sheila, and Lynn Schroeder. *Natural Birth Control*. New York: Bantam Books, 1973.

Sousa, Marion. *Childbirth at Home*. New York: Bantam Books, 1976.

Diets and Fasting

Al-Ghazzali. *The Mysteries of Fasting*. Lahore: Ashraf Press, 1968.

Bragg, Paul. *The Miracle of Fasting*. Santa Ana, Calif.: Health Science, n.d.

Ehret, Arnold. *Mucusless Diet Healing System*. Beaumont, Calif.: Ehret Publishing Company, 1922.

Gerson, Max, M.D. *A Cancer Therapy: Results of Fifty Cases*, 2d. ed. Del Mar, Calif.: Totality Books, 1975.

McKellar, Doris. *Afghan Cookery*. Kabul: Afghan Books, 1972.

New Age Vegetarian Cookbook, 4th ed. Oceanside, Calif.: The Rosicrucian Fellowship, 1973.

Newman, Laura. *Make Your Juicer Your Drug Store*. New York: Benedict Lust Publications, 1972.

Robertson, Laurel, Carol Flinders, and Bronwen Godfrey. *Laurel's Kitchen: A Handbook for Vegetarian Cookery and Nutrition*. Berkeley: Nilgiri Press, 1977.

Torre, Teofilo de la, N.D., O.D. (ed.). *Edena*, Vols. 5–8, Nos. 17–32. Santa Ana, Costa Rica: 1955–1958.

Walker, N. W. *Raw Vegetable Juices*. New York: Pyramid Books, 1970.

Yacoubi, Ahmed. *Alchemist's Cookbook: Moroccan Scientific Cuisine*. Tucson: Omen Press, 1972.

Esoteric Healing

Bailey, Alice A. *Esoteric Healing*, Vol. IV. New York: Lucis Publishing Company, 1953.

Dickinson, Martin (ed.). *The Sufi Messenger Quarterly*. Geneva: International Headquarters of the Sufi Movement, July 1970.

Gaines, Thomas. *Vitalic Breathing: The Miracle Air Discovery*. Hollywood, Calif.: Concord Press, 1947.

Heindel, Max. *Occult Principles of Health and Healing*. Oceanside, Calif.: The Rosicrucian Fellowship, 1938.

Khan, Hazrat Inayat. *The Sufi Message of Hazrat Inayat Khan*, Vol. IV. London: Barrie & Jenkins, 1961.

Healing in Afghanistan

al-Faruqi, Ismail R., Ph.D. "Moral Values in Medicine and Science." *The Journal of the IMA*, Vol. 8, Nos. 1–2. Pittsburgh, March–Sept. 1977.

Abdullah, Mawlawi, and Maulawi Ala'addin (eds.). *Mizan-ul-Tebb* (in Persian). Bombay: Haidari Press, n.d.

Akhgar, Najiba. "Popular Medical Treatments" (in Persian). *Folklore Magazine*, Vol. 3, No. 1 (June–July 1975). Kabul: Ministry of Information and Culture.

Ali, Mohammed. *The Afghans*. Kabul: Prof. Mohammed Ali, 1969.

Amin, Hamidullah. *Agricultural Geography of Afghanistan* (in Persian). Kabul: Faculty of Letters and Humanities, 1974.

Blumhagen, Rex V., M.D., and Jeanne Blumhagen, M.D. *Family Health Care: A Rural Health Care Delivery Scheme*. Wheaton, Ill.: Medical Assistance Programs, Inc., 1974.

Colvin, Diana. "Folk Medicine in Afghanistan." *Folklore Magazine,* Vol. 1, Nos. 2,3 (Aug.–Nov. 1973). Kabul: Ministry of Information and Culture.

Dupree, Louis. *Afghanistan.* Princeton: Princeton University Press, 1974.

Dupree, Nancy Hatch. *An Historical Guide to Afghanistan.* Kabul: Afghan Tourist Organization, 1971.

El-Salakawy, Ahmad A. *Spotlights on Medical Terminology: The Human Body Systems* (in Arabic). 1972.

Elkadi, Ahmad, M.D. "Professional Ethics: Ethics in the Medical Profession." *The Journal of IMA,* Vol. 7, No. 2. Pittsburgh, Sept. 1976.

Es-Salakawy, Ahmed A. *Fundamentals of Medical Terminology* (in Arabic). Dar Al Maaref, Cairo, Egypt, 1968.

Faculty of Medicine and Pharmacy. *Medical Education in Afghanistan.* Kabul: University of Kabul, 1965.

Gobar, Dr. A. H. "Narcotic Drugs Abuse Problem in Afghanistan" (in Persian). *Afghan Medical Journal,* Vol. 19, No. 1–2 (March 1975). Kabul.

Gruner, O. Cameron, M.D. *A Treatise on The Canon of Medicine of Avicenna, Incorporating a Translation of the First Book.* New York: Augustus M. Kelley, 1970.

Hunte, Pam, Mahbouba Safi, Anne Macey, and Graham Kerr. *Indigenous Fertility Regulation Methods in Afghanistan.* Kabul: Ministry of Public Health, 1975.

Kerr, Graham B., Anne Macey, Pam Hunte, Hassan Kamiab, and Mahbouba Safi. *Afghan Family Guidance Clients and Their Husbands Compared with Non-Client Neighbors and Their Husbands.* Kabul: Ministry of Public Health, 1975.

Kahn, Sayed Mohammad Husain. *Qarabādin-e Kabir* (in Persian). Bombay: Munshi Nool, publisher, n.d.

Kumorek, Martin. *Afghanistan: A Cross Cultural View.* Kabul: Peace Corps, 1976.

Levey, Martin, and Al-Khaledy. *The Medical Formulary of Al-Samarqandi and the Relation of Early Arabic Simples to Those Found in the Indigenous Medicine of the Near East and India.* Philadelphia: University of Pennsylvania Press, 1967.

Macey, Anne, Pam Hunte, and Mahbouba Safi. *The Dai: A Traditional Birth Attendant in Afghanistan.* Kabul: Ministry of Public Health, 1975.

Macey, Anne, Pam Hunte, and Hassan Kamiab. *Indigenous Health Practitioners in Afghanistan.* Kabul: Ministry of Public Health, 1975.

Mohebi, Farokhsha. "Folk Medicine" (in Persian). *Folklore Magazine,* Vol. 3, No. 1 (June–July 1975). Kabul: Ministry of Information and Culture.

Patcha, Lal. "Zadrans' Popular Medicine" (in Persian). *Folklore Magazine,* Vol. 5, No. 1 (June–July 1977). Kabul: Ministry of Information and Culture.

Rashid, Abdul, Mohammad Azam, Ahmad Jan, and Mohammad Ebrahim. *Rahat-ul-Atfal* (in Persian). Kabul: Government Printing House, Reign of Habibullah.

Sahraii, N. "Folkloric Medicine." *Folklore Magazine,* Vol. 3, No. 5 (Feb.–March 1976). Kabul: Ministry of Information and Culture.

Sameii, Dr. B. A. "Hemp and Alcohol" (in Persian). *Afghan Medical Journal,* Vol. 19, No. 1–2 (March 1975). Kabul.

Sekandar, Dr. Nasar Mohammad. *A Field Survey of Health Needs, Practices and Resources in Rural Afghanistan.* Cambridge, Mass.: Management Sciences for Health, 1975.

Stone, Russell A., Saxon Graham, and Graham B. Kerr. *Afghan Pharmacists: Their Knowledge of and Attitude toward Family Guidance.* Kabul: Ministry of Public Health, 1973.

Tabibi, Dr. Abdul H. *Sir-i Tassawf-i Afghanistan* (in Persian). Kabul: Ministry of Information and Culture, 1977.

Herbalogy

Bach, Edward. *The Twelve Healers and Other Remedies.* London: C. W. Daniel, 1975.

Christopher, Dr. John Raymond. *School of Natural Healing,* Vols. I and II. Provo, Utah: Christopher Distributing, 1975.

Culpeper, Nicholas. *Culpeper's Complete Herbal.* London: W. Foulsham & Co., Ltd, 1651.

Edinger, Philip (ed.). *How to Grow Herbs: A Sunset Book.* Menlo Park, Calif.: Lane Books, 1974.

Gonzales, Dr. Pedro Alvarez. *Yerbas Medicinales: Cómo Curarse con Plantas.* University of Mexico, Mexico City, Mexico, n.d.

Grieve, Mrs. M. *A Modern Herbal,* Vols. I and II. New York: Dover Publications, 1971.

Harper-Shove, Lt.-Col. F. *Prescriber and Clinical Repertory of Medicinal Herbs.* Bradford, England: Health Science Press, 1952.

Heffern, Richard. *The Herb Buyer's Guide.* New York: Pyramid Books, 1975.

Herb Society of America. *The Herbarist.* Boston: 1974.

Hutchens, Alma R. *Indian Herbalogy of North America.* Ontario: Merco, 1974.

Kirk, Donald R. *Wild Edible Plants of the Western United States.* Healdsburg, Calif.: Naturegraph Publishers, 1975.

Kloss, Jethro. *Back to Eden.* New York: Lancer Books, 1971.

Meyer, Joseph E., and Clarence Meyer. *The Herbalist.,* n.d.

Nature's Herb Company. *Herbs and Spices for Home Use.* San Francisco, n.d.

Pelt, J. M., and Younos, J. C., "Plantes medicinales et drogues de L'Afghanistan." Extract from *Bulletin de la Société de Pharmacie de Nancy,* No. 66 (September 1965).

Powell, Eric F., Ph.D., N.D. *The Modern Botanic Prescriber.* London: L. N. Fowler & Co., 1971.

Royal, Penny C. *Herbally Yours.* Provo, Utah: Bi-World Publishers, 1976.

Sherman, Ingrid, Ph.D., Pss.D., N.D., D.O. (GB). *Natural Remedies for Better Health.* Healdsburg, Calif.: Naturegraph Publishers, 1970.

Shook, Dr. Edward E., N.D., D.C. *Advanced Treatise on Herbology.* Mokelumne Hill, Calif.: Health Research, 1974.

Sweet, Muriel. *Common Edible and Useful Plants of the West.* Healdsburg, Calif.: Naturegraph Company, 1962.

Thomson, Samuel. *Guide to Health; or Botanic Family Physician.* Boston: J. Q. Adams, 1835.

History and Philosophy of Natural Medicine

Al-Ghazzali. *The Mysteries of Purity.* Lahore: Ashraf Press, 1970.

Bach, Edward, M.B., B.S., D.P.H. *Heal Thyself: An Explanation of the Real Cause and Cure of Disease.* London: C. W. Daniel, 1974.

Brock, J. Arthur (trans.). *Greek Medicine, Being Extracts Illustrative of Medical Writers from Hippocrates to Galen.* New York: E. P. Dutton, 1972.

Browne, E. G. *Arabian Medicine.* Cambridge: Cambridge University Press, 1962.

Haggard, Howard W., M.D. *Mystery, Magic and Medicine.* New York: Doubleday, Doran, 1933.

Hall, Manly P. *Healing: The Divine Art.* Los Angeles: Philosophical Research Society, 1971.

Khaldun, Ibn. *The Muqaddimah: An Introduction to History.* Trans. Franz Rosenthal. Princeton: Princeton University Press, 1970.

Khusrau, Amir. *Differentiation in the Fundamental and the Subsidiary Principles of Music.* Hyderabad Sind, Pakistan: Sind University Press, 1975.

Leslie, Charles. *Asian Medical Systems.* Berkeley: University of California Press, 1976.

Lindlahr, Henry, M.D. *Philosophy of Natural Therapeutics,* Vol. I. Chicago: Lindlahr Publishing Co., 1922.

Mysticism

Begg, W. D. *The Big Five of India In Sufism.* Ajmer, India: W. D. Begg, 1972.

———. *The Holy Biography of Hazrat Khwaja Muinuddin Chishti.* Tucson: The Chishti Sufi Mission of America, 1977.

de Jong-Keesing, Elisabeth. *Inayat Answers.* London: Fine Books Oriental, 1977.

Nicholson, R. A. (trans.). *Kashf Al-Mahjub of Al-Hujwiri.* London: Luzac & Co., 1970.

Schimmel, Annemarie. *Mystical Dimensions of Islam.* Chapel Hill: University of North Carolina Press, 1976.

Smith, Margaret. *Rabi'a, The Mystic, A.D. 717–801, and Her Fellow Saints in Islam.* San Francisco: The Rainbow Bridge, 1977.

Sprenger, Aloys, M.D. *Abdu-R-Razzaq's Dictionary of the Technical Terms of the Sufis.* Lahore: Zulfiqar Ahmad, 1974.
Suhrawardi, Shaikh Shahāb-Ud-Din 'Umar B. Muhammad. *The 'Awarif-Ul-Ma'arif.* Lahore: Ashraf Press, 1973.

Naturopathy, Naprapathy, Homeopathy, and Chiropractic

Airola, Paavo O., N.D. *Health Secrets from Europe.* New York: Arco Publishing Co., 1970.
———, *How to Get Well.* Phoenix: Health Plus, 1976.
Biron, W. A., B. F. Wells, and R. H. Houser. *Chiropractic Principles and Technic.* Chicago: National College of Chiropractic, 1939.
Garten, M. O., D. C. *The Health Secrets of a Naturopathic Doctor.* New York: Lancer Books, 1967.
Jensen, Bernard, D. C., N. D. *The Joy of Living and How to Attain It.* Solana Beach, Calif.: Bernard Jensen Products, 1970.
———, *The Science and Practice of Iridology.* Escondido, Calif.: Bernard Jensen, 1974.
Naprapathic Principles. Chicago: Chicago College of Naprapathy, 1942.
Pawlikowski, Timothy (ed.). *The Digest of Naprapathy/Journal of the A.T.X. Naprapathic Fraternity.* Chicago: June 1977.
Perry, Edward L., M.D. *Luyties Homeopathic Practice.* St. Louis: Formur, Inc., 1976.
Smith, Oakley. *Naprapathic Technique.* Chicago: Chicago College of Naprapathy, 1933.
Walther, David S., D.C. *Applied Kinesiology.* Pueblo: Systems DC, 1976.
Washington State Naturopathic Association, "The Reader's Health Digest." n.d.
Wendel, Paul. *Diseases of the Stomach and Intestines Naturopathic.* Brooklyn: Dr. Paul Wendel, n.d.
———. *Standardized Naturopathy.* Brooklyn: Dr. Paul Wendel, 1951.

Nutrition

Beiler, Henry G., M.D. *Food Is Your Best Medicine.* London: Neville Spearman, 1968.
Borsook, Henry, Ph.D., M.D. *Vitamins: What They Are and How They Can Benefit You.* New York: Pyramid Books, 1971.
Deal, Sheldon C., N.D., D.C. *New Life through Nutrition.* Tucson: New Life Publishing, 1974.

Heritage, Ford, B.S.M.E. Researcher. *Composition and Facts about Foods and Their Relationship to the Human Body.* Mokelumne Hill, Calif.: Health Research, 1971.

Lee Foundation for Nutritional Research. *Portfolio of Reprints for the Doctor.* Milwaukee: Lee Foundation for Nutritional Research, 1974.

Snyder, Arthur W., Ph.D. *Foods That Preserve the Alkaline Reserve.* Los Angeles: Hansen's, n.d.

Stebbing, Lionel (ed.). *Honey as Healer.* Sussex, England: Emerson Press, 1975.

Pharmacology

History of Pharmacy. New York: Parke, Davis & Company, n.d.

Huff, Barbara (ed.). *Physician's Desk Reference,* 30th ed. Oradell, N.J.: Medical Economics Company, 1976.

"Instructions to Laboratory Users," N.R. Laboratory. Chicago: Uro-Biochemical Research, 1976.

Weil, Andrew, M.D. *The Natural Mind.* Boston: Houghton Mifflin, 1972.

Wright, Harold N., M.S., Ph.D., and Mildred Montag, R.N., M.A. *A Textbook of Materia Medica Pharmacology and Therapeutics.* Philadelphia: W. B. Saunders, 1945.

Reference Works

Beaurecueil, S. de Laugier, O.P. *Manuscrits d'Afghanistan.* Le Caire, France: Imprimerie de L'Institut Français d'Archeologie Orientale, 1964.

Chen, Philip S. *Chemistry: Inorganic, Organic, and Biological.* New York: Barnes & Noble, 1968.

Compact Edition of the Oxford English Dictionary, Vols. I and II. Oxford: Oxford University Press, 1971.

DeGowin, Richard L., and Elmer L. DeGowin. *Bedside Diagnostic Examination.* New York: Macmillan, 1969.

Dunmire, John R. (ed.). *Sunset Western Garden Book.* Menlo Park, Calif.: Lane Magazine and Book Company, 1973.

Frohse, Franz, Max Brodel, and Leon Schlossberg. *Atlas of Human Anatomy.* New York: Barnes & Noble, 1970.

Gray, Henry, F.R.S. *Anatomy, Descriptive and Surgical.* Philadelphia: Running Press, 1974.

Healing Canadian Whole Earth Almanac, Vol. 2, No. 3. (Fall). Toronto, Canadian Whole Earth Research Foundation, 1971.

Holvey, David N., M.D. (ed.). *The Merck Manual of Diagnosis and Therapy,* 12th ed. Rahway, N.J.: Merck, Sharp & Dohme Research Laboratories, 1972.

Law, Donald. *A Guide to Alternative Medicine.* New York: Doubleday, 1976.

Park Seed Flowers and Vegetables, 1977. Greenwood, N.C.: 1977.

Popenoe, Cris. *Wellness.* Washington, D.C.: Yes! Inc., 1977.

Rodale, Robert (ed.). *The Encyclopedia of Organic Gardening.* Emmaus, Pa.: Rodale Books, 1971.

Steen, Edwin B., and Ashley Montagu. *Anatomy and Physiology,* Vols. I and II. New York: Barnes & Noble, 1959.

Steingass, F., Ph.D. *Persian-English Dictionary.* London: Routledge & Kegan Paul, 1963.

Wilson, John L. *Handbook of Surgery,* 4th ed. Los Altos, Calif.: Lange Medical Publications, 1969.

Windholz, Martha (ed.). *The Merck Index: An Encyclopedia of Chemicals and Drugs,* 9th ed. Rahway, N.J.: Merck & Co., 1976.

Religious and Divine Healing

Ali, A. Yusuf. *The Meaning of the Illustrious Qur'an.* Lahore: Ashraf Press, 1967.

Fox, Emmet. *The Golden Key* (pamphlet).

Gibbings, Cecil. *Divine Healing.* The Hague: East-West Publications, 1976.

Holy Bible. Cambridge: Cambridge University Press, n.d.

The Medical Group, Theosophical Research Center, London. *The Mystery of Healing.* Wheaton, Ill.: The Theosophical Publishing House, 1968.

Osborn, T. L. *Healing the Sick.* Tulsa: OSFO Publications, 1959.

Szekely, Edmond Bordeaux. *The Essene Science of Life: According to the Essene Gospel of Peace.* San Diego: Academy Books, 1975.

Zikria, Faiz A., Ph.D. (ed.). *Spiritual Dimension: Islam Ideas and Philosophy,* Vol. I. Squirrel Hill, Pa.: Zikria Bros., Inc., June 1976.

Traditional Eastern Medicine

Al-Ghazzali. *The Alchemy of Happiness.* Lahore: Ashraf Press, 1964.

A Barefoot Doctor's Manual (*The American Translation of the Official Chinese Paramedical Manual*). Philadelphia: Running Press, 1977.

Garde, R. K., M.D. *Ayurveda for Health and Long Life.* Bombay: D. B. Taraporevala Sons & Co., 1975.

Gohlman, William E. *The Life of Ibn Sina.* New York: State University of New York Press, 1974.

Khan, Hazrat Inayat. *Healing.* Tucson: Ikhwan Press, 1975.
Moss, Louis, M.D. *Acupuncture and You.* New York: Dell, 1972.
Muramoto, Naboru. *Healing Ourselves.* New York: Swan House, 1973.
Quinn, Joseph R., Ph.D. (ed.). *Medicine and Public Health in the People's Republic of China.* Bethesda, Md.: Geographic Health Studies, NIH, U.S. Dept. of HEW, 1973.
Veith, Ilza. *The Yellow Emperor's Classic of Internal Medicine.* Berkeley: University of California Press, 1973.

Unorthodox Therapies

Benjamin, Harry. *Better Sight without Glasses.* London: Health for All Publishing Company, 1929.
Brown, Arlin J. *March of Truth on Cancer,* 7th ed. Fort Belvoir, Va.: Arlin J. Brown Information Center, 1971.
Gerson, Max, M.D. *A Cancer Therapy: Results of Fifty Cases.* Del Mar, Calif.: Totality Books, 1975.
Griffin, Edward G. *World without Cancer, Parts I and II.* Westlake Village, Calif.: American Media, 1974.
Heline, Corinne. *Healing and Regeneration through Music.* Oceanside, Calif.: New Age Press, 1965.
————, *Healing and Regeneration through Color.* Oceanside, Calif.: New Age Press, 1967.
Hendren, Julie S. (publisher). *Newsreal Series.* Issue No. 4, August 1977.
Kelley, William Donald, D.D.S., M.S. *One Answer to Cancer: An Ecological Approach to the Successful Treatment of Malignancy.* Grapevine, Calif.: The Kelley Research Foundation, 1969.
Richardson, John, M.D., and Patricia Griffin, R.N. *Laetrile Case Histories: The Richardson Cancer Clinic Experience.* Westlake Village, Calif.: American Media, 1977.

Western Medicine

Goetz, John T. (ed). *Advanced First Aid and Emergency Care* (The American National Red Cross). New York: Doubleday, 1973.
Gould, George M., A.M., M.D., and Walter L. Pyle, A.M., M.D. *Anomalies and Curiosities of Medicine.* New York: Sydenham, 1937.
————. *Pocket Cyclopedia of Medicine and Surgery.* Philadelphia: Blakiston, 1926.
Vogel, Virgil J. *American Indian Medicine.* New York: Ballantine, 1973.

Index

Formulary (*cont.*):
  essence, 89
  excess of cold, 102
  excess of dryness, 102
  excess of heat, 102
  excess of moisture, 102
  fevers, 96–99
  fomentation, 89
  healing crises, 99–103
  herbal remedies, 84–93
  herbs to provoke emesis, 114–115
  humours, 103
  infusions, 89
  oil, 89–90
  oxymel, 90
  plasters, 90
  poultices, 90
  purgatives and laxatives, 110–113
  ripening biliousness, 110
  ripening of phlegm, 109–110
  salves (ointments or pomades), 90–91
  substances not ingested, 95–96
  suppositories, 91
  syrup, 90
  tinctures, 92
  water solutions, 92
  weights and measures, 81–83
Four elements (*see* Elements)
Freckles, 294
Frostbite, 295
Fruits, 47, 52
  Dried Fruit Compote, 63
  fruitarian diet, 50

Galen, xiii–xiv, 16–17, 195
Gall-bladder disorders, 66, 218–219, 226–227
Gandhi, Mahatma, 139
Gangrene, 286
Garlic, 66
Gas: excessive sex drive and, 255–256
  flatulency, 231–232
  foods for removing, 238, 242
  intestinal, 238
  stomach, 212, 221, 242
Gasping, 212
Germs, 29, 36
Gerson, Dr. Max, 74, 218, 274, 291
Giddiness and vertigo, 145
Glaucoma, 158–159
Gout, 75
Greek healers, 13–17
Grief, toxic effects, 66
Grieve, M., 85
Gripe, 237–238
Groin, hernia of, 261
Gruner, Cameron, 18, 39
Guide to Health (Thomson), 1
Gullet ailments, 182–183
  ulcers, 184, 213
Gums and teeth, 180–181

Hahnemann, Samuel, xiv, 304
Hair and nails, 281–284

baldness (alopecia), 281
care of hair, 282–283
care of nails, 283–284
Hakim Sharif ("Exalted Healer"), 3–5
Hakims, xv, 21, 39, 50, 219, 229, 242, 267
Head, 138–149
  anatomy, 140
  convulsions, 147
  delirium, 141–142
  epilepsy, 144
  eyebrow pain, 149
  forgetfulness, 145
  headaches, 139–140
  heart failure, 142
  heaviness feelings, 148
  injuries, 213
  lethargy and sleeplessness, 143
  madness, 145
  melancholy, 144
  muscular tension, 147–148
  nightmares, 143–144
  nose itching, 148–149
  paralysis, 145–146
  stiffness, 142
  trembling of limbs, 148
  vertigo and giddiness, 145
Headaches, 22, 29, 66, 139–141
  caused by hot or cold intemperament, 140
  use of cannabis sativa and narcotics, 140–141
Healing, 20–31
  body and soul form one whole unit, 20–21
  doctrine of four elements, 37–41
  doctrine of temperament, 41–44
  eleven principles of natural medicine, 21–31
  main aspects, 20–31
Healing crises, 69, 99–103
  correction of disease, 101
  signs preceding, 100
  stages, 99–100
  substances repulsed, 100–101
Health food stores, 85
Heart disease, 198–203
  anatomy, 200
  attacks, 203
  exercise for strengthening, 198–199
  fainting, 201–202
  feeling of fluid in heart area, 203
  foods to strengthen, 202
  heart attacks, 198, 203
  low-salt diets, 199
  palpitation, 300
  smoking and, 199
  stimulation of circulatory system, 199
  storehouse and seat of breath, 198
  swelling of, 202
  treatment, 198
Heart failure, 142
Heartburn, 215
Heat, 30
  caused by digestion process, 33–34
  doctrine of temperament, 42–43
  inhalations for hot imbalance, 109
  signs of excess, 102

Tuberculosis, 193, 195
Tumors: cancerous, 290–291
 skin, 289
Typhoid fever, 99

Ulcers: anus, 232
 bladder, 246
 eyes, 155
 kidneys, 243
 nose, 171
 stomach, 211–212
 testicles, 259
Ureters, 245
Urethra, 246, 250
 obstruction of, 260
Urinary bladder (*see* Bladder, urinary)
Urine, 44
 acid-alkaline range, 70–71
 burning sensation on urination, 249
 characteristics, 245–246
 inability to urinate, 250
 involuntary expulsion, 250–251
 liver ailments, 220
 mixed with blood, 251
 retention of, 249–250
 secretion of, 241
 signs of healing crisis, 101

Vaginal disorders, 264–265
 itching, 265
 secretions, 264–265
Valerian root infusion, 141, 148
Valium, 138
Vegetables, 52
 hot and cold, 47
Vegetarian diets, 53–54
Veins, broken blood vessels, 293
Vertigo and giddiness, 145
Vetch Soup, 55–56
Vibrations, 53
 of trachea, 183
Virility, lack of, 252–254
Viruses, 29
Vitality, loss of, 210
Voice, coarseness (hoarseness) of, 184
Vomiting, 114–115
 blood, 213
 causing, 212
 for conditions affecting lower parts of body, 257
 after fainting, 201
 after food is digested, 214
 healing crisis, 100
 heart palpitations and, 200

herbs to provoke emesis, 114–115
 infants, 126
 nausea and, 212
 stopping, 212

Warts, plantar, 287
Water: element, 38, 40
 essential to life, 36, 38
 liver pain after drinking, 221
 sea water, 225
 solutions, 92
 taken with food, 23
Watermelon, 107
Weakness of limbs, 146
Weights and measures, 81–83
 dry measures, 82
 equivalents between apothecary and metric systems, 82
 household measures, 83
Weil, Andrew, 141
Womb disorders, 266–267, 271–274
 boils, 272
 cancer, 273–274
 deviation of mouth of, 267
 enlarged swelling, 273
 flatulence of, 266–267
 hemorrhoids, 271
 inability to conceive, 266–267
 inclination to one side, 272
 protrusion of, 272
 strangulation of, 274
 swelling of, 272–273
 ulcers and wounds, 271
Work, moderation in, 21–23
Worms, 233
 intestinal, 239–240
Worry, toxic effects, 66
Wounds, 299–302
 bites of rabid animals, 302
 falls and blows, 299–300
 treatment of, 299

Yawning, 212
Yellow bile, 33–34
 fever, 97
 humours, 39, 103–104
 adjusting, 106–108
 compound medicines, 107–108
 single herbs to correct, 107
Yellow jaundice, 226–228
 causes, 226–227
Yoga, 139, 187, 276

Zinc deficiency, taste disorders, 170